Heather Dortch

Pg. 215 3rd ed
WC RX

SECOND EDITION

PATIENT CARE SKILLS

Documentation, Vital Signs, Bandaging,
Aseptic Techniques, Positioning, Range of Motion,
Wheelchairs, and Transfer

SECOND EDITION

PATIENT CARE SKILLS

Documentation, Vital Signs, Bandaging, Aseptic Techniques, Positioning, Range of Motion, Wheelchairs, and Transfer

Mary Alice Duesterhaus Minor, MS, PT
Scott Duesterhaus Minor, PhD, PT

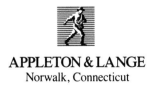

APPLETON & LANGE
Norwalk, Connecticut

0-8385-7806-3

Copyright © 1990 by Appleton & Lange
A Publishing Division of Prentice Hall
Copyright © 1984 by Reston Publishing Company, Inc.
A Prentice Hall Company

93 94 / 10 9 8 7 6

Prentice Hall International (UK) Limited, *London*
Prentice Hall of Australia Pty. Limited, *Sydney*
Prentice Hall Canada, Inc., *Toronto*
Prentice Hall Hispanoamericana, S.A., *Mexico*
Prentice Hall of India Private Limited, *New Delhi*
Prentice Hall of Japan, Inc., *Tokyo*
Simon & Schuster Asia Pte. Ltd., *Singapore*
Editora Prentice Hall do Brasil Ltda., *Rio de Janeiro*
Prentice Hall, *Englewood Cliffs, New Jersey*

Library of Congress Cataloging-in-Publication Data

Minor, Mary Alice D., 1944-
    Patient care skills : documentation, vital signs, bandaging, sterile techniques, positioning, range of motion, wheelchairs, transfer /
Mary A. Duesterhaus Minor and Scott Duesterhaus Minor. — 2nd ed.
        p. cm.
    Includes bibliographies.
    ISBN 0-8385-7806-3
    1. Transport of sick and wounded. 2. Sick—Positioning.
3. Nursing. I. Minor, Scott Duesterhaus. II. Title.
    [DNLM: 1. Nursing Care—methods. 2. Orthopedic Equipment.
3. Physical Therapy—Methods. 4. Transportation of Patients-
-methods. 5. Wheelchairs. WB 460 M666p]
RT87.T72M56 1989
610.73—dc20
DNLM/DLC
for Library of Congress   89-6741
                                                            CIP

Acquisitions Editor: Stephany S. Scott
Production Editor: Laura K. Giesman

ISBN 0-8385-7806-3

PRINTED IN THE UNITED STATES OF AMERICA

CONTENTS

Contents

CHAPTER 4

Contents

Contents

PREFACE AND ACKNOWLEDGMENTS

This manual is meant to serve as an introduction to the basic task of patient care. It is not presented as being all inclusive, but as explanatory of those tasks that are included. In addition, this manual is not presented as the final word in performing these tasks. Each of the procedures presented has alternative methods of performance. The methods included are chosen for their applicability to a variety of patients and situations. Whenever possible, alternatives and rationale are presented.

This second edition has been expanded in an effort to increase the scope of material presented. The new material encompasses documentation, bandaging and sterile techniques, vital signs, and ambulation with assistive devices through doorways. The new material covers additional basic techniques of patient care.

The most important consideration is to use the safest and most beneficial method for the patient and therapist. In some cases, this will require modification of previously learned procedures. In all cases, practice will develop safe and efficient performance.

Throughout the text we have used the term therapist. This does not mean that only physical therapists will perform these tasks. We expect that many health care workers, including physical therapist assistants, nurses, nurses' aides, and orderlies will perform these tasks. Therefore, we hope this book will be useful to many practitioners.

* * * * * * * * *

The authors wish to thank the following people for their contributions to the first edition of this text. All of this work has been successful, and is therefore retained in this second edition.

We thank Jim York and his assistants in the Department of Health, Education, Research and Development, College of Health Related Professions, Wichita State University for the photography. In addition, Jim provided advice and encouragement that was most helpful.

To Mary Edna Harrell we offer thanks and appreciation for her participation in the photography sessions, and also for her valuable suggestions. We also wish to thank Jennifer McFarland and Gary Bergner for their participation in the photography sessions.

Many thanks and much appreciation are offered to Freda Bowden, secretary in the Department of Physical Therapy, Witchita State University, for typing the original manuscript.

We wish to express our appreciation to Marvin Levand of Action Rents and Sells of Wichita for his support through the loan of equipment.

For the second edition, we wish to add our thanks to Julie Leidecker for participating in the photography sessions, to Washington University Program in Physical Therapy for the loan of equipment, and to Maryville College–St. Louis for the loan of equipment and use of facilities for photography sessions.

1
DOCUMENTATION

PURPOSE

There are many aspects of patient care, and a large number of professionals involved in the care of each patient. Coordination of these aspects and professionals requires a high level of communication among all concerned. Documentation that is precise and concise is essential in providing the level of communication required, and is thus an essential function of health care professionals.

The primary role of adequate documentation is to enhance communication for medical and legal purposes. The most important rationale for appropriate documentation is to provide the highest possible level of patient care at all times. With proper documentation, those involved with providing care for the patient and support for the patient's family will know (1) what has been determined about the patient's condition based upon interviews and tests; (2) the specific medical problems identified; (3) the goals of treatment; (4) treatment strategies to be employed; (5) the patient's response to treatment; and (6) the rationale upon which goals and treatment are based. Proper documentation also provides a valid basis for research. Without proper documentation, initial patient status and subsequent patient progress is difficult to monitor, coordination of patient care is lost, quality assurance reviews cannot be performed adequately, and reimbursement by third party payors may be compromised.

METHOD

The Problem Oriented Medical Record (POMR) System, introduced by Lawrence Weed[1], is designed to facilitate care provided to patients by organizing each medical record in a standard format. Ideally, all departments within a facility should use the same method of record keeping. This simplifies the process of communication between professionals in different departments. Even if all departments within a facility do not use the same method of record keeping, however, an individual department can implement the POMR.

A POMR is comprised of a:
1. Data base
2. Problem list
3. Initial, progress, and discharge notes.

Each medical record clearly delineates the:
1. Patient's medical history
2. Medical findings of signs, symptoms, and tests
3. Patient's problems, based upon an evaluation of signs, symptoms, and test results
4. Goals of treatment
5. Methods of treatment
6. Patient's response to treatment.

When the POMR System is fully implemented, audit for peer review and quality assurance is included. The results of audits indicate areas of strengths and weaknesses in patient care rendered, thus indicating patient outcomes requiring improvement.

PROCEDURE

Upon admission or referral, a Data Base is initiated. The Data Base includes identifying information, medical complaints voiced by the patient (symptoms), a brief medical history, and a short review of all physiological systems (signs). The information elicited from this review provides the basis for the initial Problem List, determining which health care providers need to be involved in this patient's care, and which systems require more extensive medical review.

Each problem is assigned a number and title, and is listed with the date the problem was identified when it is entered on the Problem List. Subheadings under a general problem may be used to provide more specific delineation within a major problem. Problems are often clustered under major categories: medical, psychological, and socio-economic. Any problem may be considered active, resolved, or inactive. When a problem is resolved or inactivated, the date on which this occurred is entered on the Problem List. In this way, the sequence of medical history for each patient may be maintained in an organized manner.

A medical team is comprised of all medical professionals participating in the care of an individual patient. Membership of a medical team will change as a patient's medical, psychological, and socio-economic needs change. A case manager may be any member of the medical team designated to be responsible for the overall organization of care for an individual patient. In many cases, this role is assumed by the patient's primary physician. However, any member of the medical team may identify a problem. Depending upon procedure in individual facilities, the team member identifying the problem, or the case manager, may enter a newly identified problem on the Problem List, or such entries may be made during team conferences. When a problem is resolved or inactivated, the date on which this occurred is entered on the Problem List. Again, this entry may be made by an individual team member, case manager, or during team conference, depending upon facility procedure.

FORMAT

The SOAP note format, which may be used in different approaches to medical records, is the usual format used for medical chart notes written by health care providers using the POMR System. In some facilities the SOAP note format is used without also using the data base and problem list format of the POMR System.

"S" denotes subjective data. Complaints reported by the patient and family are considered to be subjective data, and are classified as symptoms. "O" denotes objective data. Observations by health care personnel and test results are considered objective data, and are considered signs. "A" denotes assessment or analysis by the health care professional of the data included in the Subjective and Objective sections. Hypotheses concerning patient problems listed in the Assessment section are thus documented by available data, and presented for review by all members of the medical team.

Goals of treatment are also included in the Assessment section. Goals are statements of expected patient capabilities at the end of treatment, if the treatment is successful. These statements of expected outcome are based upon the results of the patient evaluation, and are written in terms that describe observable and measurable behaviors, if at all possible. Goal statements describe what the patient will be able to do. They do **not** describe what the therapist will do to the patient, or the treatment to be used with the patient.

Long term goals are statements describing functional capabilities the patient will have at the end of treatment. An example of a long term goal is:

The patient will be able to dress independently within a fifteen minute time period.

Short term goals are more discrete activities the patient will have to be able to perform to achieve the functional activities stated as long term goals. Examples of short term goals for the preceding long term goal are:

1. The patient will have functional range of motion in all joints.
2. The patient will have functional muscle strength in all major muscle groups of the upper extremity.
3. The patient will be able to weight shift from side to side and anterior/posterior while maintaining the sitting posture.

There should be a clear recognition that successful achievement of short term goals will provide the basis for successful attainment of long term goals.

"P" denotes the Plan to be followed in providing care for the specific patient. Information provided in the Plan should include (1) the priority given for treatment of each of the patient's problems; (2) an estimated timetable for meeting the patient's needs; (3) enough detail concerning treatment procedures to enable another person to continue treatment; and (4) anticipated duration of each treatment and session. The Plan should establish the actions the therapist will take in order to assist the patient in achieving the established goals.

Each section of the SOAP note need not be included in every note, however initial notes generally include all sections. Only the relevant sections are needed for any specific note. Progress notes need to include only those sections necessary for indicating changes in patient status, ie, progress or regression. Discharge notes summarize treatment provided, progress achieved, and the patient profile upon discharge. In this way, the initial status, the final status, and thus the effectiveness of therapeutic intervention can be presented in an organized manner.

REQUIREMENTS

The primary role of adequate documentation is to enhance communication for medical and legal purposes. To perform this role, documentation must be precise, concise, legible, and timely. To be precise, measurements and test results must be recorded accurately, and terminology must be used accurately and appropriately. To be concise, documentation must be organized effectively, conveying important information in a clear, unfettered fashion. To be legible, the method of note entry in a medical record should be one that allows all team members to read the entry of others accurately and without delay. Timeliness requires that notes be entered into the medical record immediately after the patient is examined or treated, in order that subsequent patient care decisions are based upon consistently and constantly updated information.

Proper grammatical usage in phrases or complete sentences should be used in all notes when prose is used. Sentences or phrases that do not contain specific information relevant to the patient's health care should not be used. Confusion and misunderstanding is avoided if abbreviations are customary and standardized within a facility. Do not assume that everyone reading a chart will interpret nonstandardized abbreviations in the same way. There are many cases in which charts or tables may be used to report individual and serial test results. The use of such charts or tables enables the communication of large amounts of information quickly, and avoids excess use of prose. Examples of such charts and tables are presented in "Evaluation Methods for the Health Professional."[2]

Periodic and consistent evaluation of patient care activities is necessary to measure and analyze the quality of patient care provided. When appropriate and significant data are reported in a consistent format, audit for peer review and quality assurance is facilitated. Records can be audited to determine if (1) actual patient care outcomes are consistent with expected patient care outcomes; and (2) patient care outcomes are dependent upon the type of treatment employed. There are several potential benefits to be gained in using audits to improve patient care rendered and patient care outcomes. A partial list of information that analysis of an audit results may yield is if:

1. Department or individual therapist treatment protocols are appropriate for the patients being treated.
2. Individual therapists are including pertinent and required information in medical chart notes.
3. Changes in department policy or protocols are necessary to improve patient care.
4. Continuing education is necessary to improve patient care skills.

Only through the availability of properly completed records can useful audits be performed.

REFERENCES

1. Weed L: *Medical Record, Medical Education, and Patient Care*, Chicago: Year Book Med., Pub, 1969.
2. Minor MAD and Minor SD: *Evaluation Methods for Health Professionals*, Reston, VA: Reston Publishing Co., 1984.

2
PREPARATION FOR PATIENT CARE

INTRODUCTION

Fundamental to all patient care are such skills as management of the environment, body mechanics, and communication. Safe implementation of a treatment procedure is best achieved when all the components of the procedure are given proper attention. Generally, a few minutes taken at the start of a procedure to plan the steps involved, and to prepare for the procedure, will increase the likelihood of safe, efficient, and effective implementation.

MANAGEMENT OF THE ENVIRONMENT

The work area is organized for the protection of the patient and staff, as well as for efficient use. Managing the environment to achieve these goals is a serious responsibility of all staff members. Some tasks may be delegated to certain personnel. However, the user is always responsible. Equipment must be returned to the proper storage place in good functioning condition. Malfunctions are to be reported in the appropriate manner to the proper person. By following these simple rules, equipment will be available and safe when needed.

Periodically, all equipment should be thoroughly inspected for wear and malfunction. Examining equipment before each use insures patient safety. Patients can, and should, be taught to inspect their equipment for wear.

When electrical equipment is used, always plug and unplug the electrical cord by holding the plug. Pulling on the cord weakens the attachment of the cord to the plug.

When equipment, such as a diathermy, is used in the treatment of a patient, position the equipment and patient to allow easy access to the patient. Should the patient need assistance quickly, improperly positioned equipment may hamper the ability to provide assistance quickly. The floor should remain uncluttered in order to avoid tripping patients and staff.

AREA PREPARATION

Prior to initiating a transfer or treatment, the bed or plinth and surrounding areas must be readied. Enough room must be allowed for unimpeded movement. Staff and patients must be able to maneuver in the area without bumping into, or tripping over, equipment. Equipment and furniture not needed during a transfer or treatment, such as an ultrasound device or mobile stool, should be moved away from the area of transfer. Besides getting in the way, many of these pieces of equipment are not stable and become dangerous if a patient tries to use them as support during a transfer.

After the area has been properly arranged, specific equipment required for the treatment may be prepared prior to beginning work with the patient. This avoids the possibility of leaving a patient unguarded or interrupting a treatment. Supplies necessary in a treatment area include linens and pillows. Plinths, mats, or beds should be prepared before the patient arrives in the treatment area. Additional sheets are used as pull sheets for transfers or for draping. Pillows for patient positioning, comfort, and safety must be within easy reach. Trying to support a patient's head while reaching for a misplaced pillow, or leaving the patient in an uncomfortable or unsafe position, is not good patient care.

BODY MECHANICS

Proper posture is required to limit stress and strain on musculoskeletal structures. When lifting, pushing, or pulling, the stresses and strains upon the musculoskeletal system are increased. Proper posture and body mechanics are based upon the alignment and functioning of the musculoskeletal system. Good body mechanics include (1) using larger and stronger muscles to perform heavy work; (2) maintaining the center of gravity of the body close to the center of the base of support; (3) keeping the combined center of gravity of the therapist and patient centered within the base of support; and (4) having a base of support that is of the appropriate size and shape.

Lifting should be initiated from a crouching or squatting position. The therapist's feet are usually placed in stride and slightly apart to widen the base of support in both the anterior/posterior and lateral directions. This negates the effects of smaller shifts in the center of gravity, and a balanced position can be more easily maintained. The trunk should be erect so that the muscles have only to maintain the erect position, and not work to extend the trunk during the lifting motion. The crouch position should be deep enough to reach the object or person to be lifted, but not so deep that the leg muscles are put at a disadvantage in regaining the upright posture.

Being as close as possible to the object or person to be lifted allows the combined center of gravity to be maintained within the base of support. Bending the hips and knees, as in a squat, allows the therapist to get close to an object, and permits lifting using strong leg muscles. When carrying patients or objects, keeping them close to the midline of the body helps maintain the combined center of gravity within the base of support.

Transfers require movements that move the center of gravity away from the center of the base of support, possibly causing a loss of balance. Increasing the size of the base of support by setting the feet in stride and slightly apart provides a larger base of support. Feet also should be free to move as the situation requires, always allowing the base of support to be reestablished under the moving center of gravity. Crossing the legs during movement should be avoided because it decreases the size of the base of support and may lead to tripping. Whenever necessary, small quick steps should be used.

When moving large pieces of equipment, such as a diathermy or parallel bars, or when guarding a patient during ambulation, position yourself facing the direction of movement in order to determine a path free from obstruction. In addition, being behind an object to be moved allows for a lifting or pushing motion, using larger muscles and body weight more efficiently.

When guarding a patient during gait training, position yourself at a 45° angle slightly to the side and rear of the patient. If the patient falls forward or backward, your position is close enough to the plane of the fall to support the patient. If the patient falls from side to side, your position will again allow support in the plane of the fall. Again, the base of support must be wide enough to support shifts in the center of gravity if the patient should start to fall. The therapist's feet should not be crossed during ambulation, nor should the therapist's feet interfere with the patient's feet or ambulatory devices.

In all cases, plan movements and prepare the area to be used before starting. Utilize proper body mechanics and safety precautions. When in doubt about your ability to lift or carry a patient or object safely, seek additional assistance.

VERBAL COMMANDS

Patients must know what they are to do and when they are to do it during transfers and treatment in order to participate effectively. Verbal commands focus the patient's attention on specifically desired actions. Instructions must be simple and in language the patient can understand in order to avoid confusion. Language used must be appropriate to the patient's level of understanding. If the patient understands medical terminology, medical terms may be used. In most cases, lay language will be required. In some cases, foreign language instructions will be necessary.

When giving commands, make them specific. Counting to "three" does not tell a patient to do anything specific. If the patient is to look up at the count of three, count to three and then say "look up." "Look up" is a specific command. It tells the patient what to do without requiring him to translate the world "three" into the specific command "look up."

The therapist should describe to the patient the general sequence of events that will occur. In addition, the patient should be instructed in his expected responses. This helps the patient to learn the skill for future independent use and increases the safety of the immediate task performance. Therefore, the therapist must determine that the patient understands the instructions. Asking the patient "Do you understand the instruction?" does not always insure understanding. Having the patient repeat the instructions in the proper order provides an opportunity for mental rehearsal of the task in addition to indicating an appropriate level of understanding.

The therapist should speak clearly and vary the tone of voice as the situation requires. Sharp commands will receive quick responses, while a soft command will elicit a slower response. Make sure the patient can hear the commands. If the patient cannot hear, or does not understand the spoken word, gestures and demonstrations may convey the necessary meaning.

PATIENT PREPARATION

For efficient use of treatment time, patient preparation should be completed prior to transport and treatment. To do so, notify nursing personnel or your department's transport personnel of preparation requirements well in advance of the scheduled treatment time. A patient should be properly dressed for transfers and treatment; this is necessary for the patient's right to modesty, for beneficial treatment, and for safety.

Hospital gowns are designed for ease in dressing and access during nursing care. They may not provide effective draping during the movements required for transfers and treatment. Properly securing the ties of a hospital gown may provide some coverage. A robe, housecoat, or two hospital gowns, one opening in front and one opening in back, may be used. If necessary, a sheet or towel may be used for draping.

Patient preparation should include dressing the patient appropriately in slacks or shorts if the lower extremities must be observed. A belt should be used as slacks or shorts will be useless or dangerous if they fall from the waist or restrict the legs. If a female patient's upper trunk must be observed, a halter top is appropriate. Shoes and socks that offer support are required if the patient is to ambulate or practice standing transfers. When a patient is dependent and working on a mat program only, slippers may be acceptable as they are easier to take off and put on as necessary. In all cases, the decision must be tempered by the patient's needs, the patient's ability to manipulate the clothing, and the requirement of the treatment.

Patients will be seen in a variety of settings. In many cases, either I.V. tubes, chest tubes, catheters, or combinations of the above will be present. When positioning, transferring, or treating patients, care must be taken not to disrupt the set-up of vital medical equipment. When chest tubes are present, there will be chest tube bottles either hung on the bed rails or taped to the floor. Care must be taken not to disturb the bottles while lowering the rails, head of the bed, or the bed itself. The bottles may hit the floor or bed, depending on their placement, before the rail, head of the bed, or bed itself is completely lowered. Breaking these bottles can be a life-threatening situation. If a chest tube bottle is broken, the chest tube should be clamped shut immediately as close to the chest as possible, and help should be requested on an emergency basis.

In all cases, tubes will limit the amount of movement available to a patient. Prior to moving the patient, or having the patient move, check the amount of movement allowed by the tubes present. Plan in advance for repositioning I.V. containers, catheter bags, oxygen masks, cannulae, and the like. This may require additional I.V. poles or posts, or another pair of hands to handle bottles while the patient is repositioned or transferred. Do not allow tubes to become tangled, pinched, kinked, stretched, or pulled out from their insertion site. Any of these occurrences will interrupt fluid or gas flow. I.V. drip rates and oxygen flow rates must not be changed. I.V. bottles must remain above the level of the patient's heart. Urinary catheter bags must remain below the level of the bladder. This is necessary to maintain the correct direction of fluid flow.

During and after transport, transfers, or repositioning, attention must be paid to appropriate draping. In many cases, even shorts or a halter top may limit observation. Draping is covering the patient with a sheet(s) or towel(s). The aim is to expose only the body segment that is necessary for treatment. The purposes of draping are to protect a patient's modesty, provide warmth, and protect wounds, scars, stumps, etc. Edges should be tucked under the patient to avoid inadvertent exposure. When repositioning a patient, advance planning is required to maintain appropriate draping during movement.

TRANSPORTING

Transporting the patient from one area to another is frequently necessary. A cart or wheelchair may be required for safety or because of hospital regulations. The patient should be transferred in an appropriate manner with proper draping during the transfers and transport. Remember to lock the brakes on the cart or wheelchair before beginning a transfer and to adjust the patient's clothing, draping, and medical accessories (I.V.'s, etc.) so they will not become tangled in the wheels or drag on the floor during transport. A mattress pad on the cart and a wheelchair cushion are used for patient comfort and protection. Additional pillows and padding are positioned for the patient's comfort and protection as necessary.

Safety belts should be used to secure the patient. There may be circumstances that require the use of restraints that the patient cannot release. If a cart has side rails, they should be used. Arms and legs should be within the cart or wheelchair so they do not get injured during transport.

VIA CART

Carts should be moved so that the patient is moving feet first, with the therapist pushing from the head of the cart. The pace should be slow and steady. Quick, jerky movements may upset a patient or make the patient nauseated. Maintain control of the cart at all times. Turn corners cautiously, and avoid bumping into walls or other objects.

VIA WHEELCHAIR

Using a wheelchair properly requires that the patient be seated well back on the seat, and that the lower extremities be placed on the footrests or legrests. Wheelchairs should also be pushed at a slow and steady pace. Quick and jerky movements can have the same effect as with a cart. Control of a wheelchair, especially when turning corners, must be maintained in the same manner as a cart.

DESCENDING CURB

To lower the wheelchair down a curb or one step, position the wheelchair so the patient is facing away from the curb. This positions the larger rear wheels at the edge of the curb to be descended. The therapist should step off the curb backwards, while facing the wheelchair.

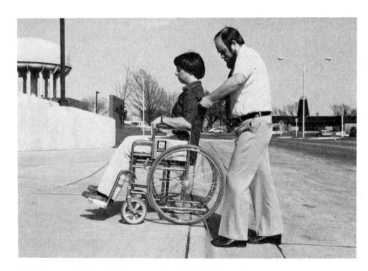

Starting position to descend curb; backward.

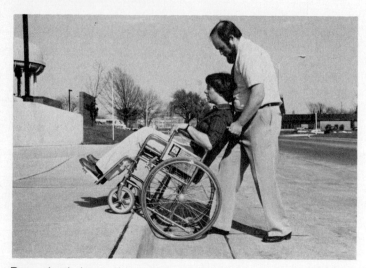

Rear wheels lowered to street.

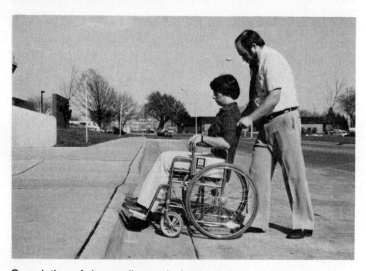

Completion of descending curb; backward.

Holding onto the handles, the therapist slowly lowers the rear wheels of the wheelchair to the street by rolling them smoothly off the edge of the curb.

Holding the handles securely, the therapist continues to roll the wheelchair backwards without allowing the front wheels to fall, until the front wheels of the wheelchair are clear of the curb. The therapist then slowly lowers the front wheels until all four wheels are securely on the lower level.

An alternative method is to approach the curb forwards. The therapist then tilts the wheelchair backwards so the front wheels are about eight inches off the ground.

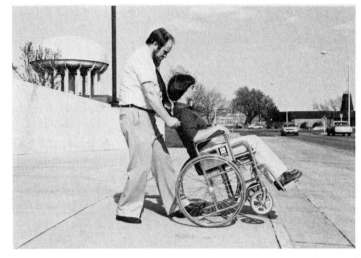

Tilting the wheelchair to descend curb; forward.

The wheelchair is then rolled slowly and smoothly off the curb onto the lower level, and then the front wheels are lowered to the ground. This method places more stress on the therapist while controlling the roll of the wheelchair over the edge of the curb.

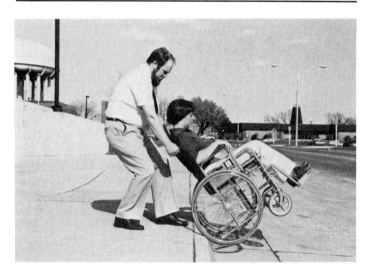

Rolling the wheelchair off the curb.

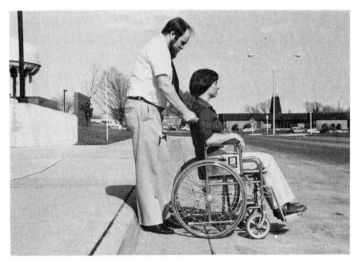

Completion of descending curb; forward.

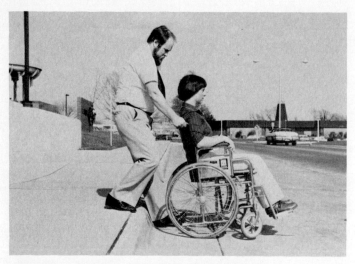

Tilting the wheelchair to ascend curb; backward.

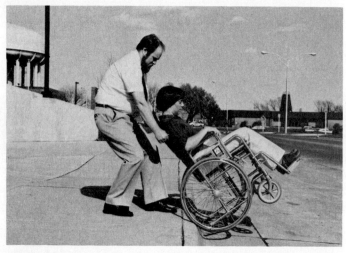

Rolling the wheelchair up the curb.

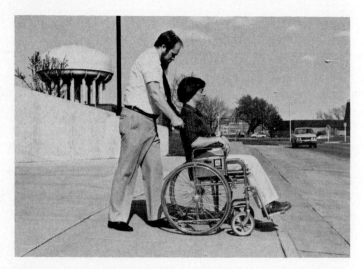

Completion of ascending the curb; backward.

ASCENDING CURB

To raise the wheelchair up a curb or one step, the foregoing procedures are reversed. The therapist tilts the wheelchair backwards onto the rear wheels.

Standing on the curb, the therapist lifts and rolls the wheelchair backwards up the curb, maintaining the backward tilt of the chair.

When all four wheels are clearly over the curb, the front wheels of the wheelchair can be lowered.

An alternative method is to approach the curb or step forwards. While facing the curb, the wheelchair is tilted backwards onto the rear wheels so the front wheels can clear the curb.

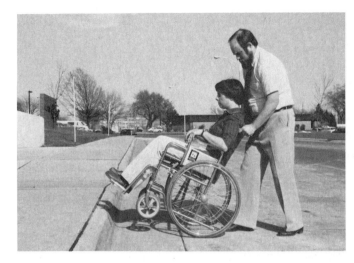

Tilting the wheelchair to ascend the curb; forward.

The wheelchair is wheeled forward, placing the front wheels on the upper level as soon as they are clearly over the upper level.

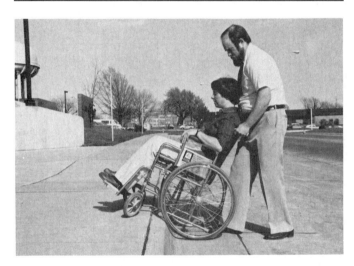

Rolling the wheelchair up the curb.

The therapist should continue to wheel the wheelchair forward until the rear wheels contact the curb. The therapist then lifts and rolls the rear wheels up and over the curb.

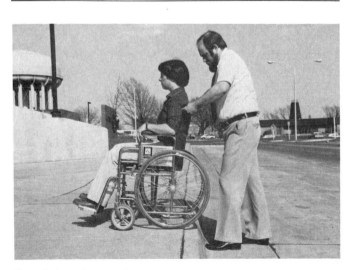

Completion of ascending the curb; forward.

DOORWAYS

The following two sections present ambulation through doorways in a wheelchair. The text and photographs depict independent ambulation. In this way, a therapist did not obscure the desired views in the photographs. Assisted ambulation through doorways in a wheelchair would be performed in the same sequence, with the therapist providing the force to open the door and propel the wheelchair.

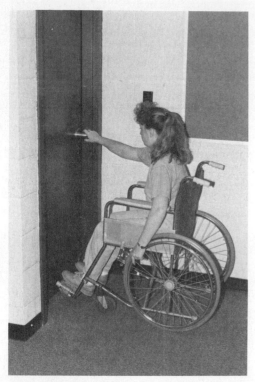

Starting position to open a door swinging away from patient.

DOOR OPENS AWAY FROM PATIENT— WITH AUTOMATIC DOOR CLOSER

The patient approaches the opening edge of the door, and grasps the doorknob.

Using a quick push, the door is opened wider than is necessary for the patient to move through the doorway. The wider opening of the door is necessitated by the fact that the door will start to close automatically.

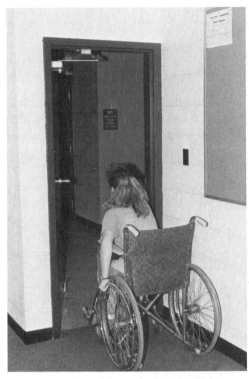

Patient opens door to prepare for passage.

The patient must move through the doorway quickly, before the automatically closing door can strike the wheelchair. Care must be taken that the door does not close and strike the patient hard enough to cause injury, or cause the patient to lose control of the wheelchair. Should the patient be unable to move through the doorway before the door closes, initially the door should only be opened partially. As the patient propels through the doorway a little at a time, the rubber bumper on the footrest closest to the hinged edge of the door is used to push the door open, and as a doorstop.

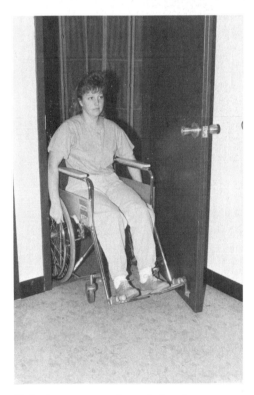

Patient progresses through the doorway.

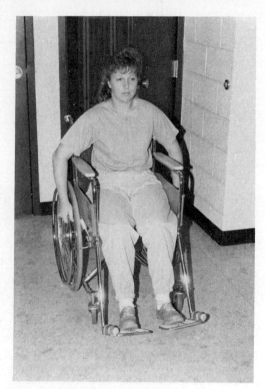

Patient completes passage through the doorway as door closes automatically.

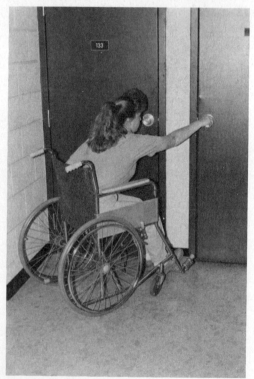

Starting position to open a door swinging toward patient.

As the patient completes moving through the doorway, the door is given one last opening push. The patient quickly propels the wheelchair out of the arc of motion of the automatically closing door, and the door is allowed to close behind the patient's wheelchair.

DOOR OPENS TOWARDS PATIENT— WITH AUTOMATIC DOOR CLOSER

The patient approaches the opening edge of the door, positioning the wheelchair outside the arc through which the door will open, facing the hinged edge of the door. The patient grasps the doorknob.

With a quick pull, the patient pulls the door open wider than is necessary for the wheelchair to pass through the doorway. The wider opening of the door is necessitated by the fact that the door will start to close automatically unless its closing is blocked by the wheelchair.

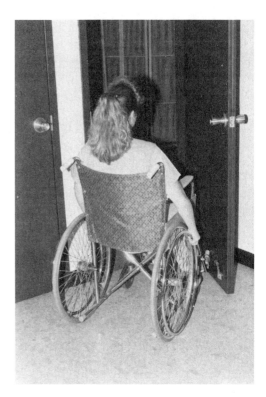

Patient blocks door to prepare for passage.

The patient must move through the doorway quickly, before the automatically closing door can strike the wheelchair. Care must be taken that the door does not close and strike the patient hard enough to cause injury, or cause the patient to lose control of the wheelchair. Should the patient be unable to move through the doorway before the door closes, the rear wheel, is used as a doorstop.

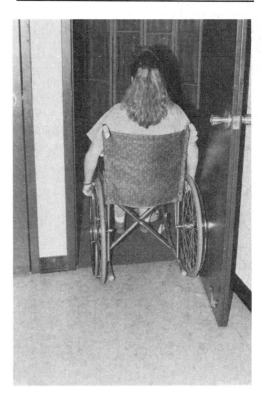

Patient progresses through the doorway.

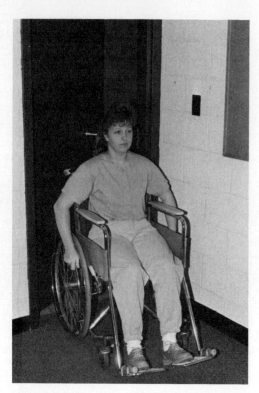

Patient completes passage through the doorway as door closes automatically.

As the patient completes moving through the doorway, the door finishes closing automatically behind the patient's wheelchair.

WITHOUT AUTOMATIC DOOR CLOSER

When the door does not have an automatic closer, rapid propulsion through the doorway is not necessary. Extra wide opening of the door is also not necessary. Propulsion of the wheelchair can be slower. Use of the wheelchair bumpers as a doorstop between the door and the patient is not required. The patient must turn to close the door, because the door will not close automatically.

WHEELIES

A wheelie is performed by balancing on the rear wheels of a wheelchair while the caster wheels are in the air. A patient must be able to perform wheelies in order to go up and down curbs when there are no curb ramps.

A wheelie begins by grasping the anterior portion of the wheel rims. A quick backward movement of the wheels places the hands in position for the forward thrust that achieves the wheelie position. The therapist must be behind the wheelchair, and must move with the wheelchair in order to guard the patient during this maneuver. The therapist's hands must always be beneath the wheelchair handles, ready to catch the wheelchair if it tilts too far backwards.

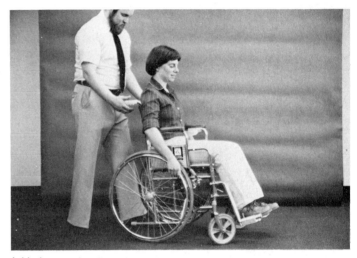

Initiating a wheelie; grasping wheel rim well forward.

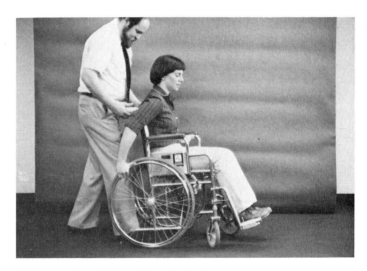

Pulling back quickly on the wheel rims.

The quick backward motion is immediately followed by a hard forward thrust on both wheels. The patient controls her balance on the rear wheels by small movements of the rear wheels.

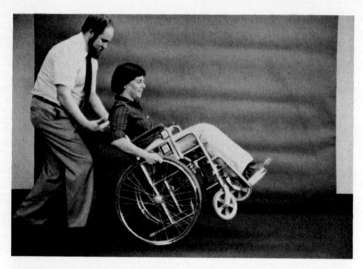

Thrusting forward into wheelie.

3
VITAL SIGNS

INTRODUCTION

Any personnel providing health care should be aware of, and able to perform simple, basic measurements of vital signs. This capability is necessary in order to monitor a patient's status at any given time during patient care, and to evaluate basic physiologic responses to treatment. The most basic vital signs monitored are pulse, blood pressure (BP), respiration, and temperature.

PULSE

PURPOSE

Pulse, or heart rate, is a noninvasive measurement used to determine how fast the heart is beating, and its regularity. Heart rate is one component of the rate–pressure product, a clinical index indicative of cardiac stress.[1] Pulse rates may be taken before, during, or following exercise. When measured during rest, the pulse rate is called the resting or basal heart rate, which is an indication of stresses placed upon the cardiovascular system at a basal metabolic level. Heart rate during exercise is indicative of the cardiovascular system's capability to provide appropriate blood flow during the stress of exercise. Heart rate measured after exercise is a measure of the cardiovascular system's recovery rate following the imposition of stress.

Pulse measurements may also be used to determine the patency of the peripheral portion of the cardiovascular system. For this purpose, presence, or lack of presence, of the pulse monitored in various sites is the most important measure, rather than heart rate. Such measurements of pulse may provide a preliminary indication of arterial occlusion resulting from physical blockage, or peripheral vascular insufficiency secondary to disease states, such as diabetes.

In addition to patency and rate, quality of pulse may provide information concerning cardiovascular status. Terms such as strong, weak, full, or thready are used to describe the quality of a pulse. A quality of pulse that varies from a normal consistent rate and strength may be indicative of disease or injury.

SITE

When taking a pulse for the purpose of measuring heart rate, the most common sites of measurement are the radial or carotid arteries.

The radial pulse is most easily palpated on the volar surface of the wrist, just medial to the styloid process of the radius.

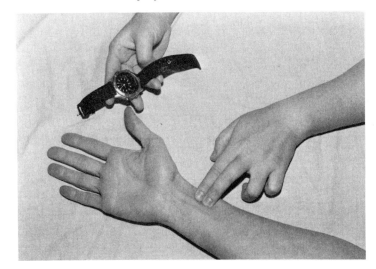

Palpation of the radial pulse.

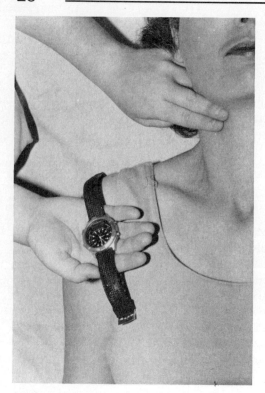

Palpation of the carotid pulse.

The carotid pulse is most easily palpated on the lateral aspect of the neck, just inferior to the angle of the mandible. Care must be taken to palpate the carotid pulse without reaching across the throat. Palpating the carotid pulse on the side of the neck, opposite to where the therapist is standing, requires the therapist to place his hand across the throat providing the potential for compromising the patient's airway.

The most common additional sites for the palpation of pulses when determining vascular patency are the brachial, femoral, popliteal, and pedal pulses. The brachial pulse may be palpated on the medial aspect of the arm, midway down the shaft of the humerus.

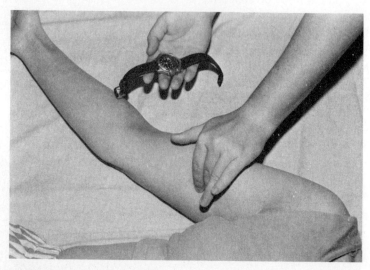

Palpation of the brachial pulse.

The femoral pulse may be palpated in the femoral triangle. Although usually a strong pulse, the femoral pulse lies deep to several large muscles, making it difficult to palpate. Care must be taken to avoid embarrassment for the patient, and pain from palpation that is too firm.

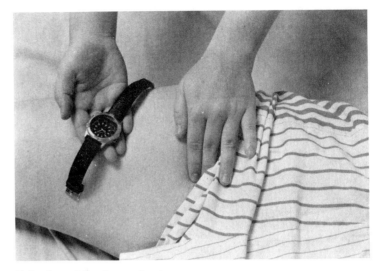

Palpation of the femoral pulse.

Both the popliteal pulse and the pedal pulse are more difficult to palpate than other pulses even in healthy patients. These pulses are most commonly susceptible to degradations of strength in patients with peripheral vascular insufficiency, making palpation more difficult. Care must be taken when palpating these pulses to avoid pressure that will obliterate the pulse.

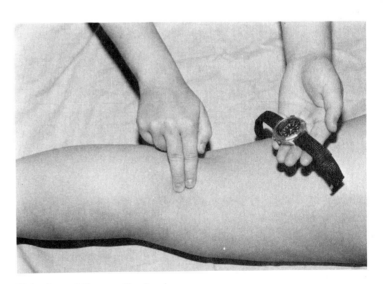

Palpation of the popliteal pulse.

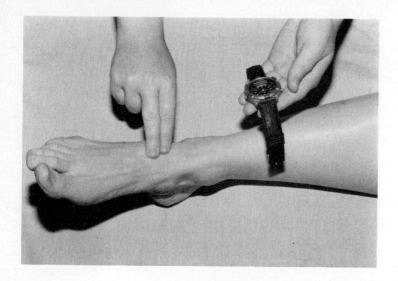

The pedal pulse may be palpated on the dorsum of the foot, approximately over the cuboid bones.

METHOD

The most common clinical method of checking pulse is manual palpation. The pads of the index and middle finger are placed over the site where the pulse is to be taken. The pad of the thumb should not be used for palpation because when taking pulse measurements, there is a pulse in the pad of the thumb. If the thumb is used for palpation, one's own pulse may be mistaken for the patient's pulse.

Care must be taken not to press too hard over the site of palpation in order to avoid obliterating the pulse and obviating the possibility of measurement. Obliteration of a pulse, even for a moderate amount of time, ie, 2 to 3 minutes, may be dangerous to a patient with an already compromised peripheral blood supply. This is especially true of the more distal pulses, which may be used when measuring peripheral vascular patency.

To obtain a heart rate in beats per minute, a watch or clock with a second hand, or a digital watch or clock that displays time in seconds may be used. Once the pulse has been palpated, beats are counted for a set period of time. The most accurate method is to count beats for a 60 second time period. The result can then be reported as heart rate in beats per minute without additional calculation. Alternative methods provide quicker results, but require additional calculation and may be less accurate.

Counting beats for a 10 second time period and multiplying the result by six, or using a 15 second time period and multiplying by four are the most common shortcuts used. These shortcuts may be less accurate than a count over a full 60 seconds. Many times, a whole number of beats does not occur within a set time period. An estimate of the fractional heartbeat is not as accurate as an exact count. Sometimes one beat in a time period is missed and not counted. In either of these cases, using a shortcut will increase the error, either sixfold or fourfold respectively.

As an example, if a patient with an actual heart rate of 72 beats per minute has a pulse taken over a 60 second time period and over a 10 second time period, an error of one beat in each method will provide two very different results. If one beat is missed during the 60 second count, the result is an error of $\frac{1}{72}$, or an error of 1.4%. For a patient with an actual heart rate of 72 beats per minute, a count over a 10 second time period should yield 12 beats. If one beat is missed during this time period, only 11 beats will be counted. This translates into a measurement of 66 beats per minute for a patient with an actual heart rate of 72 beats per minute, an error of 8.3%. Although shortcut methods are used routinely, and their results recorded without question, care must be taken to provide an accurate and valid measurement.

NORMS

Resting heart rate in adults may vary greatly, depending upon the state of physical training for each individual. The technical definition of a very slow heart rate, or bradycardia, is less than 60 beats per minute. A very fast heart rate, or tachycardia, is technically defined as a heart rate greater than 100 beats per minute. Well-trained athletes, however, may have heart rates that are considered to be indicative of bradycardia as their normal resting heart rate.[2]

Although medical literature presents various ranges of heart rates, the following ranges generally include heart rates reported in various studies. Individuals who maintain a high level of physical training may have resting heart rates from 40 to 60 beats per minute. Individuals who maintain a moderately sedentary lifestyle may have resting heart rates from 60 to 85 beats per minute. A resting heart rate greater than 85 beats per minute is usually indicative of a state of severe deconditioning for an underlying medical condition. The normal resting heart rate for infants and young children will be higher than that of adults, a range of 80 to 100 beats per minute.

Based on age, maximal heart rates are calculated for each individual. A simplified method of determining maximal heart rate, that does not take into consideration individual patient characteristics, is calculated by subtracting the patient's age from 220. Exercise that is beneficial for improving cardiovascular fitness must be performed at 70% to 90% of maximal heart rate.[3] Thus, the formula used to determine a target heart rate for cardiovascular exercise is:

$$.70 \times (220 - \text{AGE}) \text{ and } .90 \times (220 - \text{AGE})$$

Eg, the target range of heart rate for a 40-year-old person is calculated:

$$.70 \times (220 - 40) \text{ and } .90 \times (220 - 40)$$

or between 126 to 162 beats per minute.

BLOOD PRESSURE

PURPOSE

There are two primary purposes in measuring blood pressure (BP). One purpose is to determine vascular resistance to blood flow. Another purpose is to determine the effectiveness of cardiac muscle in pumping blood to overcome this vascular resistance. The two values commonly reported in measurement of BP are indications of the pressure exerted by blood against an arterial wall while the heart is in its active pumping phase (systole), and while the heart is not actively pumping (diastole). Measures of vascular resistance provide information concerning the status of different tissues and organs, and the degree that their vascular beds are constricted or dilated. Stresses placed on the heart can be initially estimated by measurement of BP. Blood pressure is also the second cardiovascular measure used for calculating the rate–pressure product.[1]

SITE

The most common site for taking BP measurements is approximately the mid-point of the shaft of the humerus. This site corresponds closely to the level of the tricuspid valve in the heart, which is considered the "reference level for pressure measurement."[2] At this level, changes in body position create minimal changes (less than 1 mm Hg) in BP measurements. Although sites other than the mid-humeral region may be used for BP measurements, such cases are rare in routine patient care.

METHOD

The most usual method of taking blood pressure is the auscultatory method. This is a non-invasive technique, utilizing a stethoscope and a sphygmomanometer. Measured in millimeters (mm), the sphygmomanometer measures the effect of pressure by raising a column of mercury (Hg). Thus, BP readings are reported by how high a column of mercury (mm Hg) has been raised while the BP measurement was being taken. An alternative instrument used for the auscultatory method is a sphygmomanometer that measures air pressure rather than a column of mercury. The results are observed on an air pressure gauge or by a digital readout.

The mercury column sphygmomanometer is usually considered a more accurate instrument. When using the mercury sphygmomanometer, care must be taken to keep the glass tube, that contains the mercury, from breaking, or the column of mercury from separating. Other alternative procedures include invasive and non-invasive methods utilizing pressure transducers and instrumentation that are technologically advanced. Such instrumentation, or training to perform invasive procedures, is not usually available to therapists, therefore, these alternative methods are not viable options.

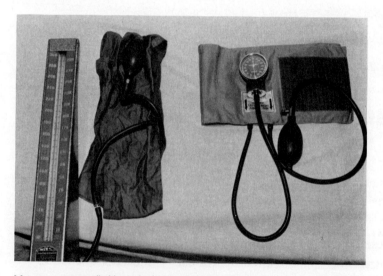

Mercury gauge (left) and air gauge (right) sphygmomanometers.

A blood pressure cuff is placed about the arm, midway between the shoulder and elbow. The antecubital arterial pulse is identified visually or by palpation.

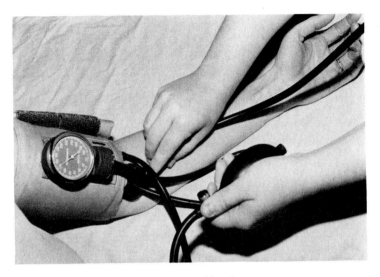

Blood pressure cuff and stethoscope in place.

A stethoscope is used to listen to the sounds of arterial blood flow through the antecubital artery in the antecubital fossa. The sounds to be monitored are called Korotkoff sounds.[2] The air relief valve on the BP pump is closed, and the BP cuff is inflated to a level well above the systolic blood pressure, approximately 200 mm Hg. As the cuff is inflated, a column of mercury rises in a graduated tube, or a gauge, increasing its pressure reading. This indicates the level of pressure exerted within the BP cuff on the arterial system.

When the cuff is inflated above the systolic BP level, the artery is totally occluded throughout the cycle, and no sounds of blood flow are heard in the antecubital artery. Air is evacuated from the cuff by opening the air relief valve slowly. As the pressure in the cuff falls below the systolic blood pressure, there is blood flow through the antecubital artery during the active pumping phase of the heart, but not during the quiet phase of cardiac activity. This difference can be identified through the stethoscope as a distinct and clear tapping sound. At this point a reading of the column of mercury, or the gauge, is taken as the value of systolic blood pressure.

As more air is evacuated from the cuff, pressure falls towards the diastolic level. When the cuff pressure is just below the diastolic blood pressure level, blood flows unimpeded through the antecubital artery during systole, and with some impediment during diastole. The distinct and clear tapping sound becomes a muffled thump at this point, when monitored through the stethoscope. A reading of the height of the column of mercury, or the gauge, is now taken as the value of diastolic blood pressure.

As air continues to be evacuated, all sounds of blood flow in the antecubital artery will cease as the cuff pressure falls approximately 5 to 10 mm Hg less than the diastolic blood pressure. At this time, the remaining air can be evacuated rapidly from the cuff by opening the air relief valve completely. The stethoscope and BP cuff may then be removed from the patient. Throughout this process, care must be taken not to maintain pressure on the antecubital artery for more than two or three minutes. If this occurs, the lack of circulation from the BP cuff occlusion may cause the patient to experience symptoms of tingling, eg, when an arm or leg ''falls asleep.''

NORMS

There are several values that may be observed or calculated when taking measurements of blood pressure. Systolic blood pressure is the first, or higher, value noted when using the auscultatory method. Diastolic blood pressure is the second, or lower, value noted when using the auscultatory method. Blood pressure readings are reported as the systolic blood pressure over the diastolic blood pressure, measured in millimeters (mm) of mercury (Hg). Thus, a patient with a systolic pressure of 120 mm Hg and a diastolic pressure of 80 mm Hg, will be reported as having a BP of 120/80 mm Hg.

The difference between the systolic pressure and the diastolic pressure is called the pulse pressure. This is the increase in pressure of arterial flow against the arterial wall caused by active pumping of the heart. The average pressure tending to push blood through the vascular system is called the mean arterial pressure. Mean arterial pressure is not a direct average of the systolic and diastolic pressures, because BP stays closer to diastolic levels during a longer portion of each heartbeat cycle. For the patient with a blood pressure of 120/80 mm Hg, the mean arterial pressure is considered to be 96 mm Hg.

Both systolic and diastolic pressures increase with age. Approximate ranges of pressure at different ages are presented in Table 1.[2]

General levels above which hypertension, and below which hypotension, are considered to exist, are presented in Table 2. It should be noted that the values in Tables 1 and 2 are general levels. Judgments based upon the values presented in Table 2 must also include a consideration of age, as presented in Table 1, and other medical information gathered upon evaluation of each individual patient.

TABLE 1. APPROXIMATE RANGES OF BLOOD PRESSURE BY AGE

	Pressure (mm Hg)		
Age	Systolic	Mean	Diastolic
Birth	85–100	75	50–65
40	125–140	110	85–100
80	160–175	125	100–115

TABLE 2. APPROXIMATE HYPERTENSION/ HYPOTENSION LEVELS (mm Hg)

Type	Hypertension Pressure	Hypotension Pressure
Systolic	140	90
Diastolic	90	60

RESPIRATION

PURPOSE

The rate and quality of respiration can be easily measured and observed, and the knowledge is useful in determining a patient's pulmonary status.

METHOD

Respiration rate and quality of respiration are measured by visual, auditory, and at times, tactile observation. In many cases, auditory observation may be performed without a stethoscope. Unobtrusive visual and auditory observations can be made just prior to, or just following, taking a pulse. In cases where shallow or quiet breathing patterns make visual and auditory observation without stethoscope difficult, a stethoscope may improve auditory observation, and tactile observation can be used.

A hand placed lightly on the patient's thorax will allow the therapist to feel the rise and fall of the chest wall during the inspiratory and expiratory phases of respiration.

An alternative method of tactile observation is to place a hand close to, but not touching or occluding, the patient's mouth and nose. Changes in the direction of air flow during respiration can be felt as slight pressure and temperature changes on the dorsal surface of the hand.

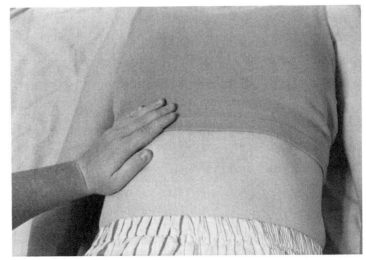

Tactile observation of respiration rate on the chest wall.

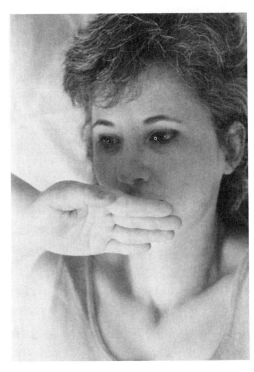

Tactile observation of respiration over the nose and mouth.

As with measuring heart rate, the number of respirations per minute is measured and recorded. Each complete respiratory cycle consists of two major phases, inspiration and expiration. Only complete respiratory cycles, those consisting of both inspiratory and expiratory phases, should be counted. Measurements may be over a 60 second time period, or shorter time periods may be used. The same problems of accuracy noted previously for determining heart rate when using shortcut methods also apply to measurements of respiration rate.

When necessary, the relative lengths of time for inspiratory and expiratory phases can be timed. A watch or clock with a second hand or a digital display of time in seconds is sufficient for these measurements. A ratio of inspiratory phase time to expiratory phase time (I/E ratio) can be calculated by using this information.

NORMS

The normal respiration rate for adults is approximately 12 breaths per minute.[2] Breathing rates at rest, less than 10 breaths per minute, or greater than 20 breaths per minute, are considered abnormal.[2] A normal breathing pattern should be even, and relatively quiet, with a slight pause between the end of expiration and the initiation of inspiration. Only a low-level hiss of air movement through the nose or mouth should be evident. Small variations may be noted, depending upon an individual's level of physical training and state of anxiety. Children normally have a respiration rate of approximately 20 breaths per minute. The normal ratio of inspiration time to expiration time within one complete respiratory cycle (I/E ratio) is normally 1:2.[4]

Following periods of exercise or during respiratory distress, respiration may increase 40 to 50 breaths per minute for short periods of time. At these times, breathing will be more shallow, and accessory muscles of respiration around the neck and shoulder region will more likely be involved in the breathing pattern. When a patient is in respiratory distress, increased sounds of respiration, termed stridor, will be evident. In patients with obstructive lung disease, an I/E ratio as high as 1:4 may be observed.[4]

TEMPERATURE

PURPOSE

Measurements of human temperature provide information concerning basal metabolic state, possible presence or absence of infection, and metabolic response to exercise. Temperature in individuals will fluctuate throughout a 24-hour period, but these fluctuations should not be more than 1°F above, or 1°F below, normal. Therapeutic treatments of heat and cold will cause variations of local site temperatures of several degrees Fahrenheit, and may affect core temperatures by 1°F or 2°F.

SITE AND METHOD

Oral, rectal, and axillary temperature measurements are most commonly used. Oral and rectal temperatures are considered the most accurate measurements of core temperature. Axillary temperature measurements are used primarily for

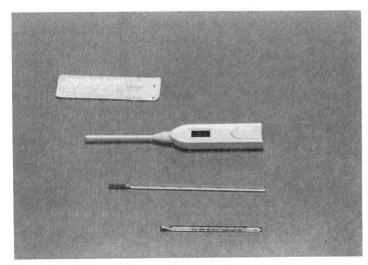

Examples of thermometers and accessories.

children, and when the patient has a medical complication that prevents easy and safe access to the mouth or rectum. All three types of thermometers are usually made of a glass tube with a bulb to hold a small quantity of mercury. Rectal thermometers have a more rounded bulb. The greater curvature is easier to insert without causing rectal discomfort. The narrower and slightly pointed end of the oral and axillary thermometers can be easier to tolerate in the mouth or axilla.

In all cases, reusable thermometers should be carefully cleansed and sterilized between uses. Prior to each use, inspection of the thermometer should be performed to determine that (1) the mercury in the thermometer has not separated, (2) the mercury in the thermometer has been shaken down to a point below the expected temperature, and (3) the glass that comprises the thermometer is not cracked, split, or chipped, and does not present any danger of cuts or mercury leakage to the patient. Many facilities now use electronic thermometers with disposable probes or probe covers. Electronic digital thermometers should have a new, unused probe cover placed over the probe before each use.

Oral temperature is taken by placing the thermometer or probe under the tongue. The tip of the thermometer or probe should be placed as far back as possible. Rectal temperature is taken by carefully inserting the thermometer into the rectum. The thermometer should be lubricated as necessary to provide comfort and safety for the patient during insertion and extraction. The thermometer should be inserted until approximately one inch of the thermometer remains exposed between the buttocks. Axillary temperature is taken by placing the tip of the thermometer into the deepest part of the axilla and lowering the arm to close the axilla over the thermometer. In all cases, the patient should remain quiet during the time a temperature measurement is being taken.

A minimum of 3 minutes is necessary for a stabile reading on a mercury thermometer. After extracting the thermometer from the measurement site, the temperature at the highest level of mercury should be read and recorded as the measurement. An electronic probe thermometer may take less time, and will signal when the highest temperature has been achieved. The digital display of temperature will hold the value of the highest temperature read until the instrument is reset.

TABLE 3. APPROXIMATE RANGES OF NORMAL TEMPERATURES

	Site			
	Oral		Rectal	
Situation	°F	°C	°F	°C
Usual normal range	96.8–99.5	36.0–37.5	96.8–99.7	36.0–37.6
Morning/Cold weather	95.0–96.8	35.0–36.0	95.9–97.0	35.3–36.1
Hard work/Emotion/A few adults/Many active children	99.7–101.0	37.6–38.3	99.7–101.5	37.6–38.6
Hard exercise			101.2–104.0	38.4–40.0

NORMS

Normal core temperature is usually considered to be 98.6° F or 37° C. This is a simplified value, however. Depending upon time of day, site of measurement, and level of activity, normal temperatures will vary within general ranges.[2] Table 3 presents temperature ranges for various situations.

Patients with a normal core temperature of 98.6° F are considered to be afebrile if their oral temperature remains below 100° F (37.8° C). If the oral temperature in these patients exceeds 100° F, they are considered to be febrile. Hypothermia occurs when rectal core temperature falls below 94° F (34.4° C). Hyperthermia occurs when rectal core temperatures rise above 106° F to 108° F (41.1° C to 42.2° C).[2] In cases of both hypothermia and hyperthermia, extremely dangerous physiological changes occur, and may result in death if not treated successfully.

REFERENCES

1. Kispert CP: Clinical measurements to assess cardiopulmonary function. *Phys Ther* 1987; 67:1886–1890.
2. Guyton AC: *Textbook of Medical Physiology*, ed 7. Philadelphia: Saunders, 1986.
3. McArdle WD, Katch FI, and Katch VL: *Exercise Physiology: Energy, Nutrition, and Human Performance*, ed 2. Philadelphia: Lea and Febiger, 1985: 358–359.
4. Humberstone N: Respiratory assessment, in Irwin S, Tecklin JS (eds): *Cardiopulmonary Physical Therapy*. St. Louis, MO: CV Mosby, 1985: vol 1, 209–229.

4
ASEPTIC
TECHNIQUES

INTRODUCTION

Increased emphasis on the importance of prevention of disease transmission and the spread of infection through proper patient care techniques has occurred in recent years. Part of this emphasis has occurred because of the increasing incidence of relatively "new" diseases, ie, Acquired Immunodeficiency Syndrome (AIDS). An expansion of research on techniques that may prevent the transmission of such diseases has also provided new information concerning cleaning, disinfecting, and sterile technique. Although the concepts of cleanliness and aseptic technique in patient care have been in use during the past two centuries, changes in these techniques are constantly occurring because of newly discovered information.

In most cases, health care personnel do not have direct contact with all steps in the sequence of preparation and use of equipment for patient care. Those who perform equipment and environment preparation are rarely involved in the use of the equipment with patients, while those who use equipment in the clinical environment during patient care are rarely involved in the process of equipment and environment preparation. It is important, however, for personnel involved in patient care to understand the underlying basis for aseptic techniques, and processes used to achieve the goals of asepsis. Use of this information makes the requirements of, and rationale for, aseptic technique and isolation precautions easier to understand, and assists in avoiding errors of omission and commission that can affect patients adversely.

Much of the material in this chapter is taken from publications in the public domain produced by the Center for Infectious Diseases, a part of the Centers for Disease Control (CDC) (Public Health Service, US Department of Health and Human Services). The Center for Infectious Diseases is continually updating recommendations for cleaning, disinfecting, and sterile technique based on an increasing body of scientific knowledge. While the information in this chapter may provide a starting point for study in aseptic techniques, it is strongly advised that updated information on specific techniques be sought directly from the Center for Infectious Diseases. Such information can be obtained from:

U S Department of Health and Human Services
Public Health Service
Centers for Disease Control
Center for Infectious Diseases
Hospital Infections Program
Atlanta, GA 30333
(404) 329-3311.

Information specific to an institution can be obtained from the appropriate department within the institution.

DEFINITIONS

ASEPTIC TECHNIQUE

Aseptic techniques consist of the methods and procedures used to create and maintain a sterile field.

BACTERIAL BARRIER

A bacterial barrier is a barrier that keeps microorganisms from coming in contact with sterile items.

CLEANLINESS

Three levels of cleanliness—cleaning, disinfection, and sterilization—have been established for equipment used in patient care.[1]

Cleaning is the physical removal of organic material or soil from objects. The process of cleaning is usually performed with water, with or without detergents. Cleaning is the least rigorous of the three levels, and is designed to remove microorganisms rather than kill them. Cleaning usually precedes either of the next two levels, disinfection or sterilization.

Disinfection is an intermediate level between cleaning and sterilization. Three levels of disinfection—high, intermediate, and low—have been defined. Disinfection is usually performed using pasteurization or chemical germicides.

Sterilization is the highest level of cleanliness. Sterilization is the destruction of all forms of microbial life by steam under pressure, liquid or gaseous chemicals, or dry heat.

CONTAMINATED

An item, surface, or field is considered to be contaminated whenever it has come into contact with anything that is not sterile.

PATIENT CARE CATEGORIES

Three categories of patient care equipment—critical, semicritical, and noncritical—[1] provide a basis for the level of cleanliness deemed necessary.

Critical items are those that are introduced directly into the circulatory system or other normally sterile areas of the body. Surgical instruments, implants, and the *bold* compartment of a hemodialyzer are examples of critical items.

Semicritical items include, but are not limited to, endotracheal tubes and fiberoptic endoscopes. There is less degree of risk of infection associated with semicritical items.

Noncritical items are items that do not touch the patient, or touch the patient in areas that are normally not sterile, ie, intact areas of skin. Blood pressure cuffs and crutches are examples of noncritical items.

RECOMMENDATIONS RANKING SCHEME

Three categories have been established to indicate the basis for recommendation by the Center for Infectious Diseases, (CDC).[2]

Category I recommendations are strongly supported by well-designed and controlled clinical studies. Recommendations in this category are considered effective, and applicable in most hospitals.

Category II recommendations are supported by highly suggestive clinical studies. Recommendations in this category may not have been adequately studied, but are based on a logical or strong theoretical rationale. Such recommendations are considered to have probable effectiveness, and as practical to implement in most hospitals.

Category III recommendations are proposed by some investigators, authorities, or organizations. At the time of classification in this category there was a lack of supporting data, strong theoretical rationale, or indication of benefits to be derived on a cost-effective basis. Recommendations in this category are considered important issues to be studied, and may be implemented by some hospitals. Such recommendations are not generally recommended for widespread use.

SHELF LIFE

Shelf life is the length of time an item that has been packaged and sterilized is considered to remain sterile as long as it remains unopened.

STERILE

An item or environment is considered sterile while there is an absence of living microorganisms.

STERILE FIELD

A sterile field is an area in which there are no microorganisms considered to be living.

UNSTERILE

Any item or environment is considered unsterile when it has not been sterilized, has come into contact with an item that is no longer considered sterile, has entered a field that is not sterile, or has exceeded its shelf life.

HANDWASHING AND SCRUBBING

PURPOSE

Many resident skin microorganisms are not highly virulent, and are not implicated in infections other than skin infections. Some of these microorganisms, however, can cause infections in patients when surgery or other invasive procedures allow them to enter deep tissues, when a patient's immunological system is severely compromised, or has an implanted device. In contrast, the transient microorganisms often found on the hands of patient care personnel can be pathogens acquired from infected patients, and may cause nosocomial infections.

The most important procedure for preventing nosocomial infections is handwashing. The initial step taken to enter a sterile field is scrubbing. Handwashing is defined as a vigorous and brief rubbing together of all surfaces of lathered hands, followed by rinsing under a flowing stream of water. Scrubbing is a series of specific steps of hand cleaning using scrub brushes and nail cleaners, and is of longer duration than handwashing.

PROCESS

Handwashing can be classified by whether plain soap or detergents, or antimicrobial containing products are used.[3] Plain soaps or detergents in bar, leaf, granule, or liquid form, suspend microorganisms in the detergent solution, allowing them to be rinsed off with water. This process is often referred to as mechanical remove of microorganisms. Use of antimicrobial containing products during handwashing kills or inhibits the growth of microorganisms. This process is often referred to as chemical removal of microorganisms.

The absolute indications for and the ideal frequency of handwashing are generally not known because of the lack of well-controlled studies. The indications for handwashing seem to depend on the type, intensity, duration, and sequence of activity. In general, superficial contact with a source not suspected of being contaminated, ie, touching an object not visibly soiled or taking a blood pressure, does not require handwashing. In contrast, prolonged and intense contact with any patient should probably be followed by handwashing. Handwashing is indicated before performing invasive procedures, taking care of particularly susceptible patients, ie, those who are severely immunocompromised or newborn infants, and *before* and *after* touching wounds. Handwashing is indicated, even when gloves are used, after situations during which microbial contamination of the hands is likely to occur, especially those involving contact with mucous membranes, blood and body fluids, and secretions or excretions, and after touching inanimate sources that are likely to be contaminated, ie, urine-measuring devices. Handwashing is an important component of the personal hygiene of all hospital personnel, and should be encouraged when personnel are in doubt about the necessity for doing so.

The circumstances that require handwashing are frequently found in high-risk units, because patients in these units are often infected or colonized with virulent or multiply-resistant microorganisms, and are highly susceptible to infection because of wounds, invasive procedures, or diminished immune function. Handwashing in these units is indicated between direct contact with different patients and is often indicated more than once in the care of one patient, eg, after touching excretions or secretions, before going on to another care activity for the same patient.

The recommended handwashing technique depends on the purpose of the handwashing. The ideal duration of handwashing is not known. For most activities, a vigorous, brief rubbing together of all surfaces of lathered hands, ie, 10 seconds, followed by rinsing under a stream of water is recommended. If hands are visibly soiled, more time may be required for handwashing.

The absolute indications for handwashing with plain soaps and detergents versus handwashing with antimicrobial-containing products are not known because of the lack of well-controlled studies comparing infection rates when such products are used. For most routine activities, handwashing with plain soap appears to be sufficient, since soap will allow most transient microorganisms to be washed off.[4-6]

Handwashing products for use in hospitals are available in several forms. It is important, however, that the product selected for use be acceptable to the personnel who will use it.[6] When plain soap is selected for handwashing, the bar, liquid, granule, or soap-impregnated tissue form may be used. It is preferable that bar soaps be placed on racks that allow water to drain. Since liquid-soap containers can become contaminated and might serve as reservoirs of microorganisms, reusable liquid containers need to be cleaned when empty and refilled with fresh soap. Completely disposable containers obviate the need to empty and clean dispensers but may be more expensive. Most antimicrobial-containing handwashing products are available as liquids. Antimicrobial-containing foams and rinses are also available for use in areas without easy access to sinks.

In addition to handwashing, personnel may often wear gloves as an extra margin of safety. As with handwashing, the absolute indications for wearing gloves are not known. There is general agreement that wearing sterile gloves is indicated when certain invasive procedures are performed or when open wounds are touched. Nonsterile gloves can be worn when hands are likely to become contaminated with potentially infective material, ie, blood, body fluids, or secretions, since it is often not known which patient's blood, body fluids, or secretions contain hepatitis B virus or other pathogens. Further, gloves can be worn to prevent gross microbial contamination of hands, ie, when objects soiled with feces are handled. When gloves are worn, handwashing is also recommended because gloves may become perforated during use and because bacteria can multiply rapidly on gloved hands.

The convenient placement of sinks, handwashing products, and paper towels is often suggested as a means of encouraging frequent and appropriate handwashing. Sinks with faucets that can be turned off by means other than the hands, eg, foot pedals, and sinks that minimize splash can help personnel avoid immediate recontamination of washed hands.

Although handwashing is considered the most important single procedure for preventing nosocomial infections, two reports showed poor compliance with handwashing protocols by personnel in medical intensive care units, especially by physicians[7] and personnel taking care of patients that are on isolation precautions.[8] Failure to wash hands is a complex problem that may be caused by lack of motivation or lack of knowledge about the importance of handwashing. It may also be caused by obstacles, ie, understaffing, inconveniently located sinks, absence of paper towels, an unacceptable handwashing product, or the presence of dermatitis caused by previous handwashing.

Scrubbing is a longer and more vigorous process than handwashing. Two classifications are recommended for scrubbing prior to entering a sterile field. The long scrub requires approximately 7 to 10 minutes. The short scrub requires approximately 3 to 5 minutes. Requirements for each type of scrub may vary from institution to institution, and institutional policy should be confirmed before it becomes necessary to scrub. Whenever there is doubt as to environmental conditions and institutional policy, assume that the long scrub is necessary.

Prior to beginning the scrubbing procedure, a freshly laundered scrub suit (pants and shirt or dress), scrub cap, and a new mask should be donned. The scrub suit should be fastened completely and properly. The scrub cap should contain all head hair and facial hair that will not be covered by a mask. The mask should be formed to fit tightly but comfortably over the nose and mouth. All facial hair not contained by the scrub cap should be covered by the mask.

Water at the scrub sink should be turned on using the knee or foot control. The temperature of the water should be warm, and the flow moderate. A preliminary wash to remove surface dirt mechanically is done by wetting and lathering both hands and arms to approximately 3 inches above the elbow. After rinsing the hands and arms, a nail cleaner from the nail cleaner dispenser is used to clean each nail on both hands. During nail cleaning, the hands are kept under the running water.

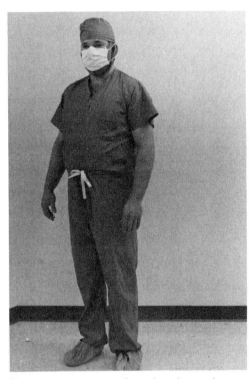

Proper arrangement of scrub suit, scrub cap, and mask.

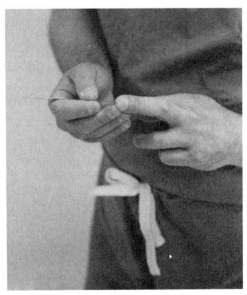

Using a finger nail cleaner.

Following completion of nail cleaning, a pre-packaged scrub sponge and brush are used. The sponge is wetted and squeezed gently to release lather. In this portion of the scrub, cleaning starts at the finger tips and moves, proximally, up each arm. In the following sequence, the sponge is used to lather the specified area, and the brush is used to scrub the area. The number of strokes listed for each segment is the minimum number, with each stroke consisting of one forward and one backward motion. Strokes should be as vigorous as tolerable for the area being cleansed. Each hand and arm must undergo the same sequence.

The fingernails of one hand are held together and given 30 strokes (short scrub—20 strokes). Each of the four long surfaces of each finger should receive 15 strokes (short scrub—10 strokes) using the narrow width of the brush.

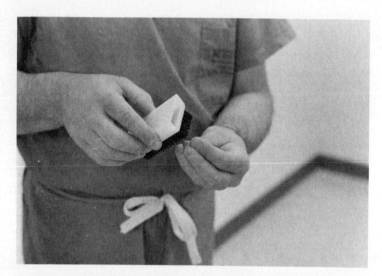

Position for fingernail scrub.

Start at one side of one hand, and clean each finger in order. Several additional strokes across each webb space should be performed as the adjacent finger surfaces are cleansed. When all fingers of one hand are completed, several additional strokes across each set of knuckles should be performed.

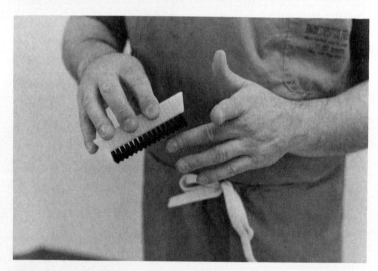

Position for finger scrub.

Each hand is considered to have six surfaces: the two narrow sides, a dorsal surface to the radial side, a dorsal surface to the ulnar side, a distal palmar surface, and a proximal palmar surface. Each surface should receive 15 strokes (short scrub—10 strokes).

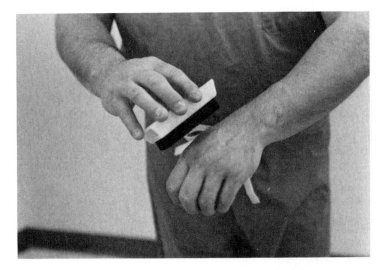

Position for hand scrub.

The forearm has four surfaces. The entire length of the forearm should not be scrubbed at one time. Starting at the wrist, scrub each of the four surfaces one third of the way up the forearm, one forearm at a time. When the forearm has been completed, several horizontal strokes across the elbow and antecubital fossa should be performed. The four surfaces of the upper arm should be scrubbed with 15 strokes (short scrub—10 strokes) to approximately 3 inches above the elbow.

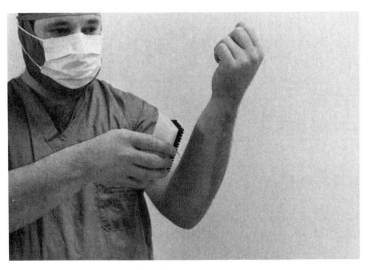

Position for forearm and arm scrub.

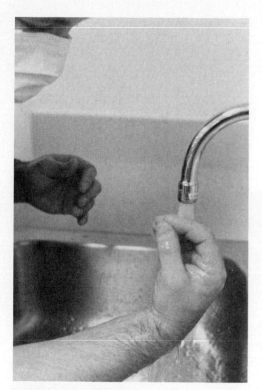

Position for scrub rinse.

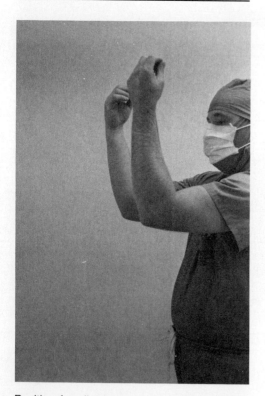

Position for allowing water run-off following scrub.

Without rinsing the first scrubbed arm, scrub the second arm. After the second arm has been scrubbed, the scrub brush and sponge are discarded. One arm at a time, rinse from fingertips to elbow, the same direction as the scrub process. After both arms have been rinsed, the arms are held in a "V" position, with the hands at shoulder height and the elbows at the lowest point. In this way, water will drip from the point of the elbows.

Having finished the scrub, the hands and arms must be protected from any contact other than a towel and gown from a sterile pack. The water should be turned off using the knee or foot control. Doors should be opened by backing into them and pushing through the doorway proceeding to the area in which the sterile pack has been opened.

Without touching the sterile field, grasp the towel from the sterile pack and lift it directly upward. The towel should be held away from the body to avoid contamination from the scrub suit. Step back from the sterile pack and let the towel open lengthwise, remaining folded in half across the width of the towel.

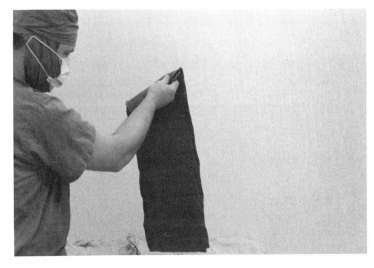

Opening a sterile towel for drying following scrub.

Using one end of the folded towel, start drying one hand and arm in the same sequence in which the scrub was performed. Dry each finger, then the hands, and then move up the forearm and arm using a slow, circular motion. Do not return to an area that has already been dried. When one arm has been completed, use the unused end of the towel to dry the other hand and arm. When drying of both arms has been completed, discard the towel without touching any other equipment or clothing.

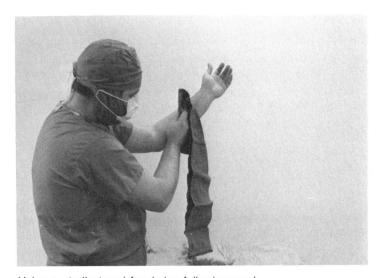

Using a sterile towel for drying following scrub.

RECOMMENDATIONS

The following are CDC (PB85-923404) recommendations for handwashing.

1. Indications
   a. In the absence of a true emergency, personnel should always wash their hands
      (1) before performing invasive procedures; *Category I*
      (2) before taking care of particularly susceptible patients, such as those who are severely immunocompromised and newborns; *Category I*
      (3) before and after touching wounds, whether surgical, traumatic, or associated with an invasive device; *Category I*
      (4) after situations during which microbial contamination of hands is likely to occur, especially those involving contact with mucous membranes, blood or body fluids, secretions, or excretions; *Category I*
      (5) after touching inanimate sources that are likely to be contaminated with virulent or epidemiologically important microorganisms; these sources include urine-measuring devices or secretion-collection apparatuses; *Category I*
      (6) after taking care of an infected patient or one who is likely to be colonized with microorganisms of special clinical or epidemiologic significance, eg, multiply-resistant bacteria; *Category I*
      (7) between contacts with different patients in high-risk units. *Category I*
   b. Most routine, brief patient care activities involving direct patient contact other than that discussed in 1.a. above, eg, taking a blood pressure, do not require handwashing. *Category II*
   c. Most routine hospital activities involving indirect patient contact, eg, handling patient medications, food, or other objects, do not require handwashing. *Category I*
2. Handwashing Technique—For routine handwashing, a vigorous rubbing together of all surfaces of lathered hands for at least 10 seconds, followed by thorough rinsing under a stream of water, is recommended. *Category I*
3. Handwashing with Plain Soap
   a. Plain soap should be used for handwashing unless otherwise indicated. *Category II*
   b. If bar soap is used, it should be kept on racks that allow drainage of water. *Category II*
   c. If liquid soap is used, the dispenser should be replaced or cleaned and filled with fresh product when empty; liquids should not be added to a partially full dispenser. *Category II*
4. Handwashing with Antimicrobial-Containing Products (Health Care Personnel Handwashes)
   a. Antimicrobial handwashing products should be used for handwashing before personnel care for newborns and when otherwise indicated during their care, between patients in high risk units, and before personnel take care of severely immunocompromised patients. *Category III* (Hospitals may choose from products in the product category defined by the FDA as health care personnel handwashes. Persons responsible for selecting commercially marketed antimicrobial health care personnel handwashes can obtain information about categorization of products from the Center for Drugs and Biologics, Division of OTC Drug Evaluation, FDA, 5600 Fishers Lane, Rockville, MD 20857.)
   b. Antimicrobial-containing products that do not require water for use, such as foams or rinses, can be used in areas where no sinks are available. *Category III*

5. Handwashing Facilities
   a. Handwashing facilities should be conveniently located throughout the hospital. *Category I*
   b. A sink should be located in or just outside every patient room. More than one sink per room may be necessary if a large room is used for several patients. *Category II*
   c. Handwashing facilities should be located in or adjacent to rooms where diagnostic or invasive procedures that require handwashing are performed, eg, cardiac catheterization, bronchoscopy, sigmoidoscopy, etc.). *Category I*

GOWNING, GLOVING, AND MASKING

Masking is performed prior to scrubbing. A fresh mask should be donned prior to each new patient encounter. The mask should be formed to fit tightly but comfortably over the nose and mouth. All facial hair not contained by the scrub cap should be covered by the mask. In addition to masks, goggles or glasses may also be considered necessary in certain situations.

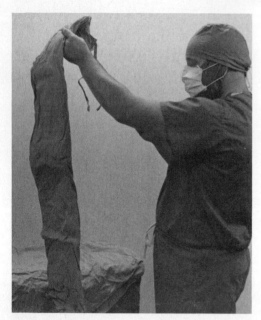

Lifting a sterile gown from sterile pack in preparation for gowning.

The gown is part of a sterile pack like the one containing the towel used for drying following the scrub process. The part of the gown facing you as you look at the sterile pack is the inside, or unsterile side. To gown, grasp the gown firmly and lift it up and away from the sterile field.

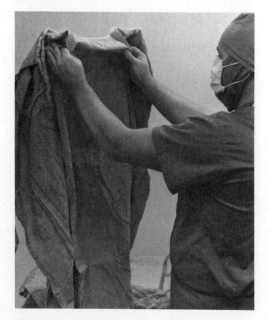

Opening a sterile gown in preparation for gowning.

Move away from the table on which the sterile pack rests. Keep hands above waist height at all times. Holding the inside of the gown only, locate the neck of the gown. Shake out the gown so it unfolds, exposing the armholes.

Without touching the outside, or sterile side of the gown, work both arms into the sleeves at the same time until hands reach the cuff of the gown. Stop when the hands reach the stockinette cuff.

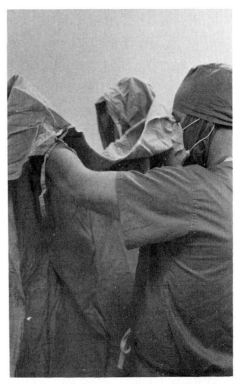

Inserting arms into armholes in a sterile gown.

Grasp the inside of the gown sleeves and have a circulating nurse or nonsterile personnel tie the inner back closure and adjust the neck closure.

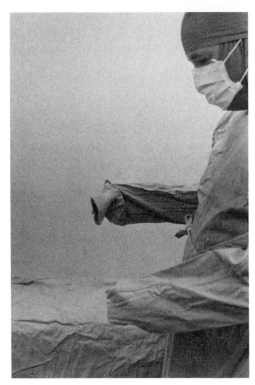

Grasping inside of sterile gown sleeves prior to gloving.

To glove, both hands must be kept inside the gown sleeves just before the stockinette cuff. Using the gown sleeves as "mittens," approach the sterile field without allowing the gown to touch the table, and open the sterile portion of the glove pack.

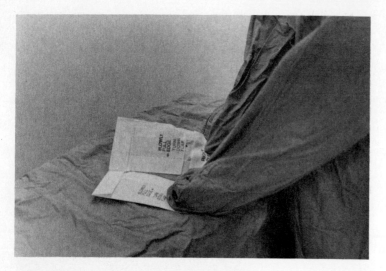

Opening inner wrapper of a sterile glove set.

Continue keeping hands inside the gown sleeves and using the gown sleeves as "mittens," and grasp the right glove with the left hand. Turn the right hand, palm up. Hook the thumb of the right hand (still inside the gown sleeve) into the thumb hole of the right-hand glove.

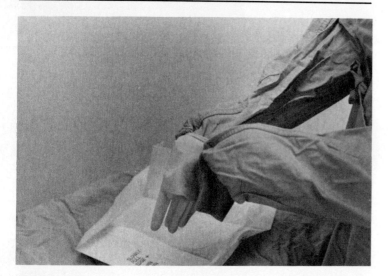

Hooking right thumb on right hand glove.

Holding the glove securely with the right thumb, work the remainder of the glove over the open end of the gown sleeve.

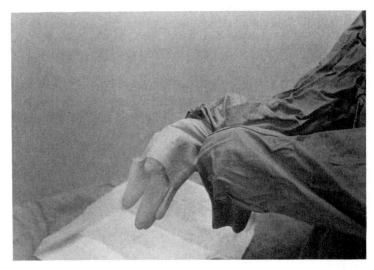

Stretching right hand glove over cuff end of sterile gown sleeve.

Once the right-hand glove has been stretched over the open end of the right-arm gown sleeve, the right hand can be worked throught the stockinette cuff of the right gown sleeve and into the right glove as if the glove were attached to the end of the sleeve in one piece.

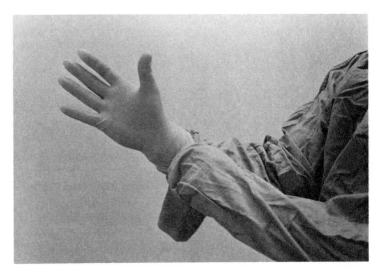

Working right hand through sterile gown sleeve into sterile glove.

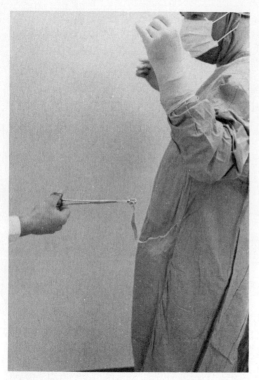

Using sterile forceps to grasp second tie on a sterile gown.

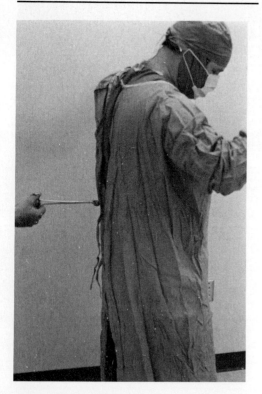

Rotating in a sterile gown to wrap second tie around back of a sterile gown.

Using the gloved right hand, pick up the left-hand glove and repeat the process to glove the left hand. Once both gloves are in place, the fingertips can be adjusted so there are no wrinkles.

If the gown is a double-tie gown, the end of the second tie will be in front of the gown. Sterile forceps should be used to grasp the end of the second tie.

The handle of the sterile forceps should be held by the circulating nurse (or nonsterile personnel) as you rotate one full turn to move the gown to cover the back and bring the second tie back to the front of the gown.

The end of the second tie is released from the sterile forceps and tied with the gloved hands in front of the gown.

An alternative method of gloving is used when only the gloved hands need to be sterile. This process may or may not be permitted in individual institutions, and procedures should be confirmed before this process is used.

The process of gowning is performed in the same manner as before, but the arms can be placed all the way through the cuffs of the gown. The sterile portion of the glove pack is then opened without touching the gloves. The wrist end of each glove has been turned back on itself, creating a cuff where the inside, or unsterile side, is now facing outward.

Grasping the right-hand glove by this cuff on the unsterile portion with a bare left hand, the right hand can be worked into the right-hand glove.

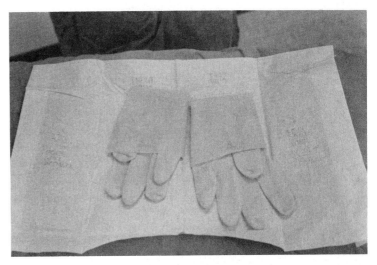

Cuffs on a sterile glove set used for alternative method of gloving.

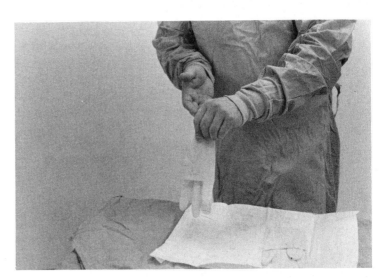

Grasping glove cuff (inside or unsterile surface) of first sterile glove to be donned for alternative method of gloving.

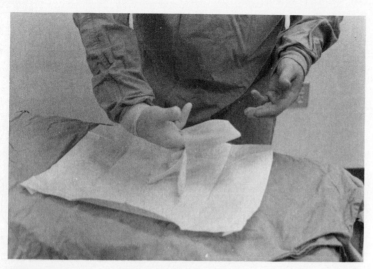

Using glove cuff (outside or sterile surface) of second sterile glove to be donned for alternative method of gloving.

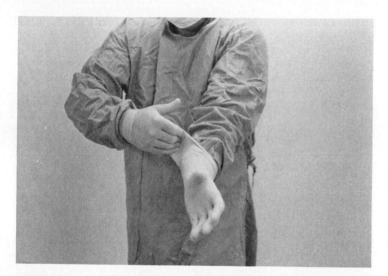

Turning the cuff over the gown sleeve in alternative method of gloving.

Once the right-hand glove is in place, it is now a sterile surface. The first two or three fingers of the gloved right hand are now slipped down inside the sterile side of the cuff of the left-hand glove, starting at the palm of the left-hand glove and pointing toward the crease of the cuff at the wrist.

The left-hand glove is then lifted using the fingers inside the cuff only. The thumb of the gloved right hand cannot be used to grasp the left-hand glove because that would cause contact with the outside of the cuff, or unsterile surface. As the left-hand glove is held by the first two or three fingers on the inside (sterile side) of the cuff, the left hand is worked into the left-hand glove.

Once the fingers of the left hand are in the proper position inside the left-hand glove, the fingers of the right hand can unfold the cuff by pulling the cuff up over the sleeve of the gown and letting the wrist portion of the glove snap into place.

The fingers of the left hand, now sterile, can now be placed on the inside (sterile side) of the right-hand glove cuff. The fingers of the gloved left hand can then unfold the cuff in the same manner as was done for the left glove. Once both glove cuffs have been properly placed, the gloves can be adjusted on the fingers.

STERILE FIELD

The primary goal of using aseptic techniques is to provide and maintain a sterile field. A sterile field is most commonly required in an operating room. There may be a necessity for a sterile field, however, in patient care areas other than the operating room for the performance of minor procedures. Such procedures may include, but not be limited to, insertion of arterial lines or debridement of burn patients.

Eight guidelines for providing and maintaining a sterile field are presented on the following pages. The first four concern the creation of a sterile field. The second four concern the maintenance of the sterile field.

GUIDELINE 1

All items used within the boundaries of a sterile field must be sterile. The items must have been properly sterilized and maintained to preserve their sterile state. Once items have been sterilized, they must be used within the allowable shelf life of the item and sterilization process. The expiration date, or end of shelf life is marked on each sterile package. Certain types of equipment and different types of packaging may affect the shelf life of a sterile package.

It should be clearly understood that a shelf life date is not a guarantee of a sterile package. Packages are only considered to remain sterile if the: (1) initial packaging was done properly; (2) initial sterilization was done properly; (3) package was stored in a proper manner and not mishandled during storage; and (4) shelf life date has not been exceeded.

GUIDELINE 2

Once a sterile container or package has been opened, the edges are not considered sterile. Care in opening sterile packages is required to avoid having the edges touch the contents of the package, or having the edges touch the gloved hands or sterile gown. Most sterile packages have enough packaging material around the edges to keep the unsterile edges far enough away from the sterile contents.

Whenever possible, single-use items are preferred. Because single-use items are discarded after the initial use, they cannot become contaminated before they are reused. This does not mean, however, that they cannot become contaminated before the initial use through improper technique or carelessness.

GUIDELINE 3

Gowns are considered to be sterile in the front from shoulder level to table top level, including the sleeves. It is for this reason that during and after scrubbing, gowning, and gloving, the hands must be maintained above waist level, in front of the body, and that nonsterile personnel can only assist with tie ends by using sterile forceps.

GUIDELINE 4

Tables are only considered to be sterile at table top level. Sterile drapes may cover the top of a surface and descend on all sides of the surface. Such draping may be on the patient or on the instrument table. In all cases, only the top surface is considered sterile. Demarcation of sterile surfaces are fairly easy on tables, but more difficult on patients. A guideline to use for demarcation on a patient that is draped is to consider that a surface above the level of the instrument table, or above waist level, whichever is higher, is a sterile surface as long as it is properly draped. Undraped, improperly draped surfaces, or surfaces below the top of the instrument table or waist, should be considered unsterile.

GUIDELINE 5

Only sterile persons and items may enter a sterile area, and only sterile persons and items may touch other sterile items without causing contamination. Non-sterile personnel may not touch any item in a sterile area or any item to be placed in a sterile area. Transfer of sterile items into a sterile area may be accomplished by using sterile forceps to hold the item as it is passed into the sterile area and then the set of forceps is considered contaminated after a single use, and may not be used again until properly sterilized. In addition, nonsterile personnel may not reach across a sterile field or into a sterile area.

GUIDELINE 6

Activity in a sterile area cannot be allowed to render the area unsterile. Sterile personnel may not leave and reenter a sterile area without performing the scrubbing and gowning process again. Sterile personnel should not sit on, or lean against, unsterile surfaces. Movements within the sterile area must be measured and careful to avoid contact between sterile and unsterile surfaces.

All personnel, sterile or unsterile, in or around a sterile area must be aware of the boundaries of the sterile area. Any contamination of the sterile area must be pointed out immediately for the protection of the patient.

GUIDELINE 7

Penetration of a sterile barrier must be considered to have contaminated the sterile field. Liquids are the most likely cause of penetration of a sterile barrier. The type of material used will have an affect on the usefulness of a sterile barrier. Carelessness in the disposal of liquids within a sterile field may also cause penetration of a sterile barrier if the liquids are spilled on the barrier.

A less noticable, but highly potential cause of penetration is air flow. The design of climate control for sterile areas should provide for the most purified air possible, and a slightly higher gradient of air pressure in the sterile area. The higher air pressure gradient in the sterile area will cause air flow away from the site of potential infection. The climate control system should also be physically separated from other areas of the institution so that airborne micro-organisms picked up in sterile areas do not permeate the atmosphere of the entire institution.

GUIDELINE 8

If there is doubt about the sterility of an area, a field, or an item, it should be considered unsterile. Improper packaging, sterilization processing, storage, or handling may occur without overt signs. Appropriate use of all items in a sterile environment is the responsibility of the user. Only cautious judgment, rigid discipline, and appropriate use can provide the best patient safety.

Sterile areas and fields should be prepared as close to the time of use as feasible. They should not be left unattended. Sterile fields should not be prepared and then covered for later use. A delay in use necessitates the preparation of a new sterile field.

DRESSINGS

PURPOSE

The purposes of wound dressings are to (1) physically protect the site of injury; (2) prevent contamination of the wound; (3) prevent transmission of infection from the wound; and (4) promote healing. Protection from further injury requires that a wound be physically protected. Transmission of infection both to the patient and from the patient is limited by the practice of appropriate aseptic techniques and the application of appropriate dressings. Healing is promoted by protecting the wound and with the use of appropriate antimicrobial agents.

There is little definitive research concerning specific clinical protocols for wound dressings. Many institutions and health care professionals have preferred methods of caring for specific types of wounds. This section presents basic information concerning wound dressings. Information for a specific institution should be sought from the appropriate departments or practicioners within the institution.

EVALUATION

Documentation of wound characteristics is necessary for appropriate selection of dressing materials and protective agents, and for monitoring progress in wound healing. Evaluation of the wound is necessary to determine (1) the cause of the wound; (2) location, area, and depth of the wound; (3) if the wound is wet or dry; and (4) if the wound is infected, and if infected, the source and mechanism of infection; and microorganism of infection.

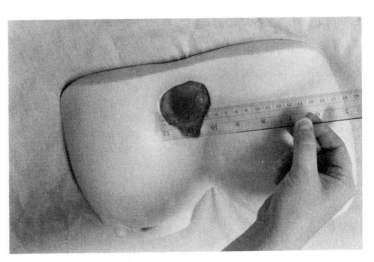

Measurement of a wound.

Measurement of the wound can be performed using a standard ruler. The ruler should not make contact with the wound itself.

Another method of documenting the extent of a wound is by photographing the wound.

TYPES AND PROCEDURES

The first step in applying a dressing is to gather the necessary supplies. Gauze pads, roll gauze, tape, and topical agents should be within easy reach. Sterile fields, when required, should be set up in the proper manner. All preparations should be performed in accordance with established guidelines.

Protection of the wound from contamination requires the appropriate application of aseptic techniques. In this regard, correct handwashing procedures before and after each patient contact is one of the most important measures that an individual can take. Proper masking, gowning, gloving, and sterile field techniques, when indicated, will limit the potential of introducing infection into a clean wound. Proper disposal of soiled dressing materials will limit the potential of transmitting infectious material from a contaminated wound.

Choice of materials for, and method of application of, dressings may depend upon (1) the cause of the wound; (2) whether the wound is clean or contaminated, and if contaminated the microorganism causing the contamination; (3) the type, if any, of an antimicrobial agent to be applied; (4) the site, area, and depth of the wound; and (5) whether a trained professional, the patient, or the patient's family will be responsible for monitoring and changing the dressing.

In most cases, the soft dressings used for purposes 2 to 4 listed in the first section under "DRESSINGS" will provide adequate physical protection for the site of injury. On occasion, a rigid dressing will be used to immobilize the site of injury. Immobilization may be necessary to maintain approximation of different aspects of the injury site.

Because of existing knowledge about the effects of specific medications on specific microorganisms, identification of the specific microorganism responsible for infection is beneficial in treating any wound. Specific antimicrobial agents may require specific types of dressing materials to insure that the agent is properly applied to the wound. Additional information concerning underlying pathologic conditions of the patient will also aid in wound treatment.

Four types of dressing applications are generally used: 1. Dry to dry; 2. Wet to wet; 3. Wet to dry; and 4. Occlusive. A dry to dry dressing is the application of dry absorbent or nonabsorbent dressing to cover the wound. A wet to wet dressing is the application of a gauze pad soaked in normal saline solution or other similar solution before application. Resoaking of the wet dressing is done while the dressing remains in place to keep the dressing from drying out, and becoming embedded in the eschar. The wet to wet dressing also assists in softening the eschar in preparation for removal. A wet to dry dressing is the application of a wet dressing that is allowed to dry before removal. The dressing dries embedded in the eschar, and acts to debride the wound when the dried, embedded dressing is removed. Occlusive dressings are applied to provide a semi-permeable barrier to air and moisture penetration.

If a wound is draining, absorption of exudate may be a consideration requiring a dry dressing. If a wound tends to be dry, and the dryness impedes healing, a wet dressing would be required. Limiting exposure to air, or maintaining a moist environment within the wound, may require an occlusive dressing.

The location of a wound may dictate the type of dressing applied, or the method of application. Dressings over joints may have to be rigid to prevent joint motion from disrupting the efficiency of the dressing, or may have to be applied in a way that accommodates joint motion. Wounds may require extensive modification of bedding arrangements and seating arrangements so sleeping and sitting activities do not disrupt the dressing or put pressure on the wound. The depth of a wound may require additional measures, such as packing the wound, to insure that the deeper layers of a wound heal before the surface layers to avoid the development of an unhealed cavity.

Underlying pathologic conditions may have an impact on the dressings chosen and the application of dressings. No dressing, unless specifically designed to do so in an emergency situation, should ever be applied in a manner that impedes blood circulation. The existence of peripheral vascular disease, such as accompanies diabetes, is a condition that requires special attention to avoid further impairment of circulation.

If long term care of a wound is required, care may be provided outside an institutional setting if appropriate. Careful evaluation and consideration must be given to the patient's or the family's capability to understand and carry-out specific instructions. Patient or family care of wounds and dressings may dictate, or be dictated by, the complexity of the care required. A wound site that cannot be easily seen by the patient is not a wound that can be cared for by a patient. Physical or mental impairment of the patient, ie, a stroke which impairs manual dexterity or Alzheimer's disease, which impairs mental faculties, may prohibit a patient from providing wound care, even if the wound site is visible. If non-institutional care is considered appropriate, the patient or patient's family must be carefully instructed in proper wound care. Whenever possible, simple procedures should be used.

The most basic dressing is an adhesive strip of tape with a small gauze center, commonly called by the trademark name Band-Aid. These dressings are available from a number of companies in various shapes and sizes. Topical antimicrobial agents may be applied underneath the gauze portion of this dressing. The adhesive portion of the dressing may be regular plastic, or may be a less dense plastic or paper with a hypoallergenic adhesive to limit skin reaction to the application of the dressing. Dressings with non-adhering pads that do not stick to wounds or the exudate from wounds are also available. These dressings, often called by the trademark name Telfa Pads, are also available from a number of companies in various shapes and sizes. These basic dressings are usually best for small wounds, although self-made dressings of the same nature can be constructed in any size if the necessary material is available. The size of these dressings, whether prepackaged or constructed, should cover the wound site plus some portion of healthy tissue on all sides of the wound. In no case should the adhesive portion of the dressing come in contact with the wound itself.

Gauze is the most common material used for dressings, and is available in pads and rolls. Sterile and nonsterile gauze is available in several sizes. If sterile gauze is to be used, proper aseptic handling techniques should be used during opening and application. Dressings constructed from gauze may use topical antimicrobial agents underneath the dressing if required.

The gauze can then be unrolled directly onto the skin in a continuous motion. In all cases, the amount of pressure applied to the gauze during wrapping should not be excessive in order to avoid impairing circulation.

A spiral wrap is applied by wrapping gauze in a continuous manner around the limb segment. The free end of a roll of gauze is placed on the limb segment. The roll is angled slightly to accommodate for the sloping contour of the limb segment to be wrapped.

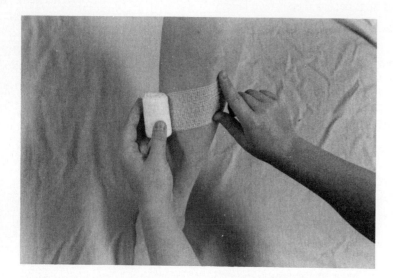

Gauze pads are usually secured by tape or a gauze roll. Gauze rolls are generally applied in a spiral wrap or in a "figure-of-eight" wrap. It is usually easiest to apply a gauze wrap by laying the portion of the gauze roll that is unwrapping against the limb segment to be wrapped, with the still rolled gauze away from the limb segment.

Proper position of roll gauze in preparation for a gauze dressing wrap (spiral or figure-of-eight).

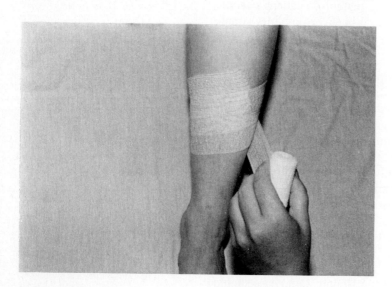

The roll of gauze is then unrolled around the limb segment in the amount deemed necessary. Each successive wrap should overlap the previous wrap by about half.

Spiral wrap (partially completed).

A figure-of-eight wrap is started in the same manner as a spiral wrap. Rather than a continuous wrap in the same direction, however, the direction of wrapping is changed each time the gauze completes one loop of the figure-of-eight. A sample sequence, starting in a medial direction on the lower leg would be:

1. In a medial direction across the anterior aspect of the leg;
2. Around the medial aspect of the leg;
3. Across the posterior aspect of the leg in a medial to lateral direction;
4. Around the lateral aspect of the leg and across the anterior aspect of the ankle;
5. Around the medial aspect and under the foot;
6. Up over the lateral aspect of the foot and across the anterior aspect of the ankle in a lateral to medial direction;
7. Around the medial aspect of the leg to the posterior aspect of the leg; and
8. Around the posterior aspect of the leg in a medial to lateral direction.

These steps are repeated in various combinations of directions around the leg, ankle, and foot. The edges of the gauze roll should overlap by about half. Eventually all necessary aspects of the lower leg, ankle, and foot should be covered. The result is a figure-of-eight wrap.

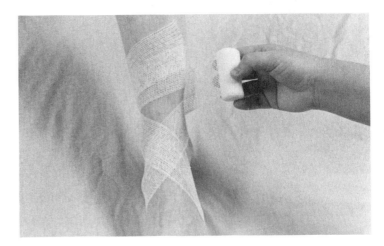

Figure-of-eight wrap (partially completed).

Tape may be cloth adhesive tape, or paper tape which has a hypoallergenic adhesive. Tape may be cut to the required length with scissors or torn from the roll. Tape is torn by unrolling the desired amount and firmly grasping the tape between the pad of the thumb and the side of the index finger of each hand, with the hands approximately 1 inch apart.

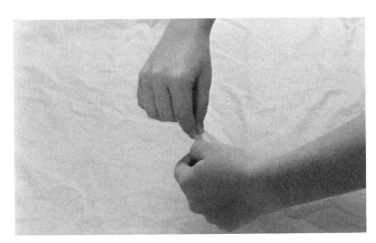

Position for tearing tape.

Care should be taken not to roll the edges of the tape over because this makes the tape harder to tear. A quick movement of one hand away from the body and the other hand towards the body will cause the tape to tear between the two hands. Even cloth adhesive tape can be torn in this manner as long as the edges have not been rolled over.

Because tearing or cutting tape usually takes two hands, it may be more efficient to tear several pieces before applying the wrap or dressing. The pieces can be hung from the edge of a table, cabinet, or bed frame by sticking only a small portion of one end to the table, and letting the remainder of the piece hang free. The pieces should be hung in an accessible place since one hand is usually required to secure the dressing or wrap while the tape is applied. If tape is applied circumferentially on a limb segment, the ends should not overlap. Adhesive and paper tape do not have enough elasticity to avoid impairment of circulation if the ends overlap in this situation.

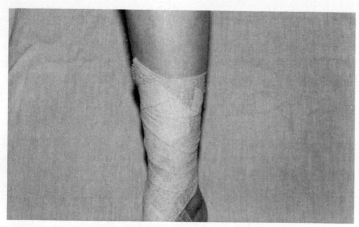

Proper use of a circumferential piece of adhesive tape. Ends do not overlap.

Compression wraps are applied to control edema by using elastic material, most commonly called by the trademark name ACE Wraps. The material is usually available in 3, 4, 5, and 6 inch widths. Compression wraps are also applied in spiral or figure-of-eight wraps. When applying compression wraps, more pressure is applied distally than proximally. This provides for compression on edematous segments without constricting the flow of fluid towards the core of the body for subsequent elimination. Frequent examination of compression wraps is necessary to insure that the amount of compression applied is appropriate, and that the wrap remains in place.

The entire limb segment distal to the top most edge of the wrap must be covered by the wrap with appropriately graded pressure.

CLEANSING

PURPOSE AND PROCESS

It is neither necessary nor possible to sterilize all patient care items. Institutional policies can identify whether cleaning, disinfecting, or sterilization of an item is indicated to decrease the risk of infection, or transmission of infection. The process used with any item depends upon its intended use. Any microorganism, including bacterial spores, that come in contact with normally sterile tissue can cause infection. Thus, it is important that all items that will touch normally sterile tissues be sterilized. It is less important that objects touching mucous membranes be sterile. Intact mucous membranes are generally resistant to infection by common bacterial spores but are not resistant to many other microorganisms, such as viruses and tubercle bacilli; therefore, items that touch mucous membranes require a disinfection process that kills all but resistant bacterial spores. In general, intact skin acts as an effective barrier to most microorganisms; thus, items that touch only intact skin need only be clean.

Items must be thoroughly cleaned before processing, because organic material, eg, blood and proteins, may contain high concentrations of microorganisms. Also, such organic material may inactivate chemical germicides and protect microorganisms from the disinfection or sterilization process. For many noncritical items, blood pressure cuffs or crutches, cleaning can consist only of (1) washing with a detergent or a disinfectant-detergent; (2) rinsing; and (3) thorough drying.

Steam sterilization is the most inexpensive and effective method for sterilization. Steam sterilization is unsuitable, however, for processing plastics with low melting points, powders, or anhydrous oils. Items that are to be sterilized but not used immediately need to be wrapped for storage. Sterility can be maintained in storage for various lengths of time, depending on the type of wrapping material, the conditions of storage, and the integrity of the package.

Several methods have been developed to monitor steam sterilization processes. One method is to check the highest temperature that is reached during sterilization and the length of time that this temperature is maintained. In addition, heat- and steam-sensitive chemical indicators can be used on the outside of each pack. These indicators do not reliably document sterility, but they do show that an item has not accidentally bypassed a sterilization process. As an additional precaution, a large pack might have a chemical indicator both on the outside and the inside to verify that steam has penetrated the pack.

Because ethylene oxide gas sterilization is a more complex and expensive process than steam sterilization, it is usually restricted to objects that might be damaged by heat or excessive moisture. Before sterilization, objects also need to be cleaned thoroughly and wrapped in a material that allows the gas to penetrate. Chemical indicators need to be used with each package to show that it has been exposed to the gas sterilization process. Ethylene oxide gas is toxic and precautions, eg, local exhaust ventilation, should be taken to protect personnel.[9] All objects processed by gas sterilization also need special aeration according to manufacturers' recommendations before use to remove toxic residues of ethylene oxide.

Powders and anhydrous oils can be sterilized by dry heat. Microbiological monitoring of dry heat sterilizers and following manufacturers' recommendations for their use and maintenance usually provides a wide margin of safety for dry heat sterilization.

Liquid chemicals can be used for sterilization and disinfection when steam, gas, or dry heat sterilization is not indicated or available. With some formulations, high-level disinfection can be accomplished in 10 to 30 minutes, and sterilization can be achieved if exposure is for significantly longer times. Nevertheless, not all formulations are equally applicable to all items that need to be sterilized or disinfected. No formulation can be considered as an ''all purpose'' chemical germicide. In each case, more detailed information can be obtained from the EPA, descriptive brochures from the manufacturers, peer-review journal articles, and books.

Gloves may be indicated to prevent skin reactions when some chemical disinfectants are used. Items subjected to high-level disinfection with liquid chemicals need to be rinsed in sterile water to remove toxic or irritating residues and then thoroughly dried. Subsequently, the objects need to be handled aseptically with sterile gloves and towels and stored in protective wrappers to prevent recontamination.

Hot-water disinfection (pasteurization) is a high-level, nontoxic disinfection process that can be used for certain items, eg, respiratory therapy breathing circuits.

In recent years, some hospitals have considered reusing medical devices labeled disposable or single use only. In general, the primary, if not the sole, motivation for such reuse is to save money. Since there is lack of evidence indicating increased risk of nosocomial infections associated with reusing *all* single-use items, a categorical recommendation against all types of reuse is not considered justifiable. Rather than recommending for or against reprocessing and reuse of all single-use items, it appears more prudent to recommend that hospitals consider the safety and efficacy of the reprocessing procedure of each item or device separately and the likelihood that the device will function as intended after reprocessing. In many instances it may be difficult if not impossible to document that the device can be reprocessed without residual toxicity and still function safely and effectively. Few, if any, manufacturers of disposable or single-use medical devices provide reprocessing information on the product label.

Hydrotherapy pools and immersion tanks present unique disinfection problems in hospitals. It is generally not economically feasible to drain large hydrotherapy pools that contain thousands of gallons of water after each patient use. Typically, these pools are used by a large number of patients and are drained and cleaned every 1 to 2 weeks. The water temperature is typically maintained near 37°C. Between cleanings, water can be contaminated by organic material from patients, and high levels of microbial contamination are possible. One method to maintain safe pool water is to install a water filter of sufficient size to filter all the water at least 3 times per day and to chlorinate the water so that a free chlorine residual of approximately 0.5 mg/L is maintained at a pH of 7.2 to 7.6. Local public health authorities can provide consultation regarding chlorination, alternate halogen disinfectants, and hydrotherapy pool sanitation.

Hubbard and immersion tanks have entirely different problems than large pools, since they are drained after each patient use. All inside surfaces need to be cleaned with a disinfectant-detergent, then rinsed with tap water. After the last patient each day, an additional disinfection step is performed. One general procedure is to circulate a chlorine solution (200 to 300 mg/L) through the agitator of the tank for 15 minutes and then rinse it out. It is also recommended that the tank be thoroughly cleaned with a disinfectant-detergent, rinsed, wiped dry with clean cloths, and not filled until ready for use.

An alternative approach to control of contamination in hydrotherapy tanks is to use plastic liners and create the "whirlpool effect" without agitators. Such liners make it possible to minimize contact of contaminated water with the interior surface of the tank and also obviate the need for agitators that may be very difficult to clean and decontaminate.

RECOMMENDATIONS

The following are CDC (PB85-923404) recommendations for cleansing.

1. Cleaning.
   All objects to be disinfected or sterilized should first be thoroughly cleaned to remove all organic matter (blood and tissue) and other residue. *Category I*
2. Indications for Sterilization and High-Level Disinfection
   a. Critical medical devices or patient-care equipment that enter normally sterile tissue or the vascular system or through which blood flows should be subjected to a sterilization procedure before each use. *Category I*
   b. Laparoscopes, arthroscopes, and other scopes that enter normally sterile tissue should be subjected to a sterilization procedure before each use; if this is not feasible, they should receive at least high-level disinfection. *Category I*
   c. Equipment that touches mucous membranes, eg, endoscopes, endotracheal tubes, anethesia breathing circuits, and respiratory therapy equipment, should receive high-level disinfection. *Category I*
3. Methods of Sterilization
   a. Whenever sterilization is indicated, a steam sterilizer should be used unless the object to be sterilized will be damaged by heat, pressure, or moisture or is otherwise inappropriate for steam sterilization. In this case, another acceptable method of sterilization should be used. *Category II*
   b. Flash sterilization [270°F (132°C) for 3 minutes in a gravity displacement steam sterilizer] is not recommended for implantable items. *Category II*
4. Biological Monitoring of Sterilizers
   a. All sterilizers should be monitored at least once a week with commercial preparations of spores intended specifically for that type of sterilizer, ie, *Bacillus stearothermophilus* for steam sterilizers and *Bacillus subtilis* for ethylene oxide and dry heat sterilizers. *Category II*
   b. Every load that contains implantable objects should be monitored. These implantable objects should not be used until the spore test is found to be negative at 48 hours. *Category II*
   c. If spores are not killed in routine spore tests, the sterilizer should immediately be checked for proper use and function and the spore test repeated. Objects,

other than implantable objects, do not need to be recalled because of a single positive spore test unless the sterilizer or the sterilization procedure is defective. *Category II*

   d. If spore tests remain positive, use of the sterilizer should be discontinued until it is serviced. *Category I*

5. Use and Preventive Maintenance—Manufacturers' instructions should be followed for use and maintenance of sterilizers. *Category II*

6. Chemical Indicators—Chemical indicators that will show a package has been through a sterilization cycle should be visible on the outside of each package sterilized. *Category II*

7. Use of Sterile Items—An item should not be used if its sterility is questionable, eg, its package is punctured, torn, or wet. *Category I*

8. Re-processing Single-Use or Disposable Items

   a. Items or devices that cannot be cleaned and sterilized or disinfected without altering their physical integrity and function should not be re-processed. *Category I*

   b. Re-processing procedures that result in residual toxicity or compromise the overall safety or effectiveness of the items or devices should be avoided. *Category I*

Different types of microorganisms require different levels of disinfection.

Different objects and equipment may be cleansed and stored in different ways, depending upon the level of criticality.

These charts are reproduced from the Guideline For Handwashing and Hospital Environmental Control, 1985 (PB85-923404), produced by the Center for Infectious Diseases, CDC. For application in clinical settings, updated information from the CDC, and information specific to the institution, should be sought.

TABLE 1. LEVELS OF DISINFECTION ACCORDING TO TYPE OF MICROORGANISM

| Levels | Bacteria Tubercle | | Fungi* | | Viruses | |
	Vegetative	Bacillus	Spores		Lipid and Medium size	Non-lipid and small
High	+ +	+	+ ′	+	+	+
Intermediate	+	+	± §	+	+	± ″
Low	+	−	−	±	+	−

* Includes asexual spores but not necessarily chlamydospores or sexual spores.

⁺ Plus sign indicates that a killing effect can be expected when the normal use-concentrations of chemical disinfectants or pasteurization are properly employed; a negative sign indicates little or no killing effect.

± Only with extended exposure times are high-level disinfectant chemicals capable of actual sterilization.

§ Some intermediate-level disinfectants can be expected to exhibit some sporicidal action.

″ Some intermediate-level disinfectants may have limited virucidal activity.

TABLE 2. METHODS OF ASSURING ADEQUATE PROCESSING AND SAFE USE OF MEDICAL DEVICES

Object and Classification	Example	Method	Comment
Patient Care Objects			
Critical			
Sterilized in the hospital	Surgical instruments and devices; trays and sets	1. Thoroughly clean objects and wrap or package for sterilization. 2. Follow manufacturer's instructions for use of each sterilizer or use recommended protocol. 3. Monitor time-temperature charts. 4. Use commercial spore preparations to monitor sterilizers. 5. Inspect package for integrity and for exposure of sterility indicator material before use. 6. Use before maximum safe storage time has expired if applicable.	Sterilization processes are designed to have a wide margin of safety. If spores are not killed, the sterilizer should be checked for proper use and function; if spore tests remain positive, discontinue use of the sterilizer until properly serviced. Maximum safe storage time of items processed in the hospital varies according to type of package or wrapping material used; follow manufacturer's instructions for use and storage times.
Purchased as sterile	Intravenous fluids; irrigation fluids; normal saline; trays and sets	1. Store in safe, clean area. 2. Inspect package for integrity before use. 3. Use before expiration date if one is given. 4. Culture only if clinical circumstances suggest infection related to use of the item.	Notify the Food and Drug Administration, local and state health departments, and CDC if intrinsic contamination is suspected.
Semi-critical			
Should be free of vegetative bacteria. May be subjected to high-level disinfection rather than sterilization process	Respiratory therapy equipment and instruments that will touch mucous membranes	1. Sterilize or follow a protocol for high-level disinfection. 2. Bag and store in safe, clean area. 3. Conduct quality control monitoring after any important changes in the disinfection process.	Bacterial spores may survive after high-level disinfection, but these usually are not pathogenic. Microbiologic sampling can verify that a high-level disinfection process has resulted in destruction of vegetative bacteria; however, this sampling is not routinely recommended.
Non-critical			
Usually contaminated with some bacteria	Bedpans; crutches; rails; ECG leads	1. Follow a protocol for cleaning or, if necessary a low-level disinfection process.	
Water-produced or treated	Water used for hemodialysis fluids	1. Assay water and dialysis fluids monthly. 2. Water should not have more than 200 bacteria/mL and dialysis fluids not more than 2000 bacteria/mL.	Gram-negative water bacteria can grow rapidly in water and dialysis fluids and can place dialysis patients at risk of pyrogenic reactions or septicemia. These water sources and pathways should be disinfected routinely.

WASTE DISPOSAL

PURPOSE AND PROCESS

There is no epidemiologic evidence to suggest that most hospital waste is any more infective than residential waste. Moreover, there is no epidemiologic evidence that hospital waste disposal practices have caused disease in the community. Therefore, identifying wastes for which special precautions are indicated is largely a matter of judgment about the relative risk of disease transmission. Aesthetic and emotional considerations may override the actual risk of disease transmission, particularly for pathology wastes.

Since a precise definition of infective waste that is based on the quantity and type of etiologic agents present is virtually impossible, the most practical approach to infective waste management is to identify those wastes that represent a sufficient potential risk of causing infection during handling and disposal and for which some special precautions appear prudent. Hospital wastes for which special precautions appear prudent include microbiology laboratory waste, pathology waste, and blood specimens or blood products. The risk of either injury or infection from certain sharp items, eg, needles and scalpel blades, contaminated with blood also needs to be considered when such items are disposed of. While any item that has had contact with blood, exudates, or secretions may be potentially infective, it is not normally considered practical or necessary to treat all such waste as infective. CDC has published general recommendations for handling infective waste from patients on isolation precautions.[10] Additional special precautions may be necessary for certain rare diseases or conditions such as Lassa Fever.[11] The EPA has published a draft manual (Environmental Protection Agency. Office of Solid Waste and Emergency Response. Draft Manual for Infectious Waste Management, SW-957, 1982. Washington, 1982) that identifies and categorizes other specific types of waste that may be generated in some research-oriented hospitals. In addition to the above guidelines, local and state environmental regulations may also exist.

Solid waste from the microbiology laboratory can be placed in steam-sterilizable bags or pans and steam sterilized in the laboratory. Alternatively, it can be transported in sealed, impervious plastic bags to be burned in a hospital incinerator. A single bag is probably adequate if the bag is sturdy (not easily penetrated) and if the waste can be put in the bag without contaminating the outside of the bag; otherwise, double-bagging is indicated. All slides or tubes with small amounts of blood can be packed in sealed, impervious containers and sent for incineration or steam sterilization in the hospital. Exposure for up to 90 minutes at 250°F (121°C) in a steam sterilizer, depending on the size of the load and type container, may be necessary to assure an adequate sterilization cycle.[12,13] After steam sterilization, the residue can be safely handled and discarded with all other non-hazardous hospital solid waste. All containers with more than a few milliliters of blood remaining after laboratory procedures and/or bulk blood may be steam sterilized, or the contents may be carefully poured down a utility sink drain or toilet.

Disposables that can cause injury, such as scalpel blades and syringes with needles, should be placed in puncture-resistant containers. Ideally, such containers are located where these items are used. Syringes and needles can be placed intact directly into the rigid containers for safe storage until terminal treatment. To prevent needle-stick injuries, needles should not be recapped, purposely bent, or broken by hand. When some needle-cutting devices are used, blood may be aerosolized or spattered onto environmental surfaces. However, there is not any data currently available from controlled studies examining the effect, if any, of the use of these devices on the incidence of needle-transmissible infections.

It is often necessary to transport or store infective waste within the hospital prior to terminal treatment. This can be done safely if proper and common-sense procedures are used. The EPA draft manual mentioned contains guidelines for the storage and transport of infective waste, both on-site and off-site.

RECOMMENDATIONS

The following are CDC (PB85-923404) recommendations for disposal of infective, or potentially infective, waste.

1. Identification of Infective Waste
   a. Microbiology laboratory wastes, blood and blood products, pathology waste, and sharp items (especially needles) should be considered as potentially infective and handled and disposed of with special precautions. *Category II*
   b. Infective waste from patients on isolation precautions should be handled and disposed of according to the current edition of the "Guideline for Isolation Precautions in Hospitals." (This recommendation is not categorized since the recommendations for isolation precautions are not categorized.)
2. Handling, Transport, and Storage of Infective Waste
   a. Personnel involved in the handling and disposal of infective waste should be informed of the potential health and safety hazards and trained in the appropriate handling and disposal methods. *Category II*
   b. If processing and/or disposal facilities are not available at the site of infective waste generation, ie, laboratory, etc, the waste may be safely transported in sealed impervious containers to another hospital area for appropriate treatment. *Category II*
   c. To minimize the potential risk for accidental transmission of disease or injury, infective waste awaiting terminal processing should be stored in an area accessible only to personnel involved in the disposal process. *Category III*
3. Processing and Disposal of Infective Waste
   a. Infective waste, in general, should either be incinerated or should be autoclaved prior to disposal in a sanitary landfill. *Category III*
   b. Disposable syringes with needles, scalpel blades, and other sharp items capable of causing injury should be placed intact into puncture-resistant containers located as close to the area in which they were used as is practical. To prevent needle-stick injuries, needles should not be re-capped, purposely bent, broken, or otherwise manipulated by hand. *Category I*
   c. Bulk blood, suctioned fluids, excretions, and secretions may be carefully poured down a drain connected to a sanitary sewer. Sanitary sewers may also be used for the disposal of other infectious wastes capable of being ground and flushed into the sewer.
   Category II (Special precautions may be necessary for certain rare diseases or conditions such as Lassa fever.[10])

LAUNDRY

PURPOSE AND PROCESS

Although soiled linen has been identified as a source of large numbers of pathogenic microorganisms, the risk of actual disease transmission seems to be negligible. Therefore, rigid rules and regulations for hygienic storage and processing of clean and soiled linen are not required or recommended.

Soiled linen can be transported in the hospital by cart or linen chute. If linen chutes are used, bagging of linen is necessary. Improperly designed linen chutes can be a means of transmission of microorganisms throughout an institution if bagging of linen is not done.[14]

Soiled linen may or may not be sorted in the laundry before being loaded into washer/extractor units. Sorting before washing protects both machinery and linen from the effects of objects in the linen and reduces the potential for re-contamination of clean linen that sorting after washing requires. Sorting after washing minimizes the direct exposure of laundry personnel to infective material in the soiled linen and reduces airborne microbial contamination in the laundry. Protective apparel and appropriate ventilation can minimize these exposures.

The microbicidal action of the normal laundering process is affected by several physical and chemical factors.[15] Although dilution is not a microbicidal mechanism, it is responsible for the removal of significant quantities of micro-organisms. Soaps or detergents loosen soil and also have some microbicidal properties. Hot water provides an effective means of destroying microorganisms, and a temperature of at least 71°C (160°F) for a minimum of 25 minutes is commonly recommended for hot-water washing. Chlorine bleach provides an extra margin of safety. A total available chlorine residual of 50 to 150ppm is usually achieved during the bleach cycle. The last action performed during the washing process is the addition of a mild acid to neutralize any alkalinity in the water supply, soap, or detergent. The rapid shift in pH from approximately 12 to 5 also may tend to inactivate some microorganisms.

Satisfactory reduction of microbial contamination can be achieved at lower water temperatures of 22 to 50°C when the cycling of the washer, the wash formula, and the amount of chlorine bleach are carefully monitored and controlled.[16,17] Instead of the microbicidal action of hot water, low-temperature laundry cycles rely heavily on the presence of bleach to reduce levels of microbial contamination. Regardless of whether hot or cold water is used for washing, the temperatures reached in drying and especially during ironing provide additional significant microbicidal action.

RECOMMENDATIONS

The following are CDC (PB85-923404) recommendations for handling of soiled and clean laundry.

1. Routine Handling of Soiled Linen
   a. Soiled linen should be handled as little as possible and with minimum agitation to prevent gross microbial contamination of the air and of persons handling the linen. *Category II*

(1) All soiled linen should be bagged or put into carts at the location where it was used; it should *not* be sorted or pre-rinsed in patient care areas. *Category II*

(2) Linen soiled with blood or body fluids should be deposited and transported in bags that prevent leakage. *Category II*

    b. If laundry chutes are used, linen should be bagged, and chutes should be properly designed. *Category II*

2. Hot-Water Washing—If hot water is used, linen should be washed with a detergent in water at least 71°C (160°F) for 25 minutes. *Category II*

3. Low-Temperature Water Washing—If low temperature (<70°C) laundry cycles are used, chemicals suitable for low-temperature washing at proper-use concentration should be used. *Category II*

4. Transportation of Clean Linen—Clean linen should be transported and stored by methods that will ensure its cleanliness. *Category II*

HOUSEKEEPING

PURPOSE AND PROCESS

Although microorganisms are a normal contaminant of walls, floors, and other surfaces, these environmental surfaces rarely are associated with transmission of infections to patients or personnel. Therefore, extraordinary attempts to disinfect or sterilize these environmental surfaces are rarely indicated. Routine cleaning and removal of soil, however, are recommended.

Cleaning schedules and methods vary according to the area of the hospital, type of surface to be cleaned, and the amount and type of soil present. Horizontal surfaces, eg, bedside tables and hard-surfaced flooring, in patient care areas are usually cleaned on a regular basis, when soiling or spills occur, and when a patient is discharged. Cleaning of walls, blinds, and curtains is recommended only if they are visibly soiled. Disinfectant fogging is an unsatisfactory method of decontaminating air and surfaces and is not recommended.

There is no epidemiologic evidence to show that carpets influence the nosocomial infection rate in hospitals.[18] Carpets, however, may contain much higher levels of microbial contamination than hard-surfaced flooring and can be difficult to keep clean in areas of heavy soiling or spillage. Therefore, appropriate cleaning and maintenance procedures are indicated.

Disinfectant-detergent formulations registered by the EPA can be used for environmental surface cleaning, but the actual physical removal of microorganisms by scrubbing is probably as important, if not more so, than any antimicrobial effect of the cleaning agent used. Therefore, cost, safety, and acceptability by housekeepers can be the main criteria for selecting any such registered agent. The manufacturers' instructions for appropriate use should be followed.

Special precautions[19] for cleaning incubators, mattresses, and other nursery surfaces with which neonates have contact must be followed, since inadequately diluted solutions of phenolics used for such cleaning and poor ventilation have been associated with hyperbilirubinemia in newborns.[20]

RECOMMENDATIONS

The following are CDC (PB85-923404) recommendations for housekeeping.

1. Choice of Cleaning Agent for Environmental Surfaces in Patient Care Areas— Any hospital-grade disinfectant-detergent registered by the EPA may be used for cleaning environmental surfaces. Manufacturers' instructions for use of such products should be followed. *Category II*
2. Cleaning of Horizontal Surfaces in Patient Care Areas
   a. Uncarpeted floors and other horizontal surfaces, eg, bedside tables, should be cleaned regularly and if spills occur. *Category II*
   b. Carpeting should be vacuumed regularly with units designed to filter discharged air efficiently, cleaned if spills occur, and shampooed whenever a thorough cleaning is indicated. *Category II*
3. Cleaning Walls, Blinds, and Curtains—Terminal cleaning of walls, blinds, and curtains is not recommended unless they are visibly soiled. *Category II*
4. Disinfectant fogging—Disinfectant fogging should not be done. *Category I*

ISOLATION

RATIONALE AND BASIS

ELEMENTS

Spread of infection within a hospital requires three elements:

1. Source of infecting organisms;
2. Susceptible host; and
3. Means of transmission for the organism.

SOURCE

The source of the infecting agent may be patients, personnel, or on occasion, visitors, and may include persons with acute disease, persons in the incubation period of the disease, or persons who are colonized by the infectious agent but have no apparent disease. Another source of infection can be the person's own endogenous flora, or autogenous infection. Other potential sources are inanimate objects in the environment that have become contaminated, including equipment and medications.

HOST

Patients' resistance to pathogenic microorganisms varies greatly. Some persons may be immune to or able to resist colonization by an infectious agent; others exposed to the same agent may establish a commensal relationship with the infecting organism and become asymptomatic carriers; still others may develop clinical disease. Persons with diabetes mellitus, lymphoma, leukemia, neoplasia, granulocytopenia, or uremia and those treated with certain antimicrobials, corticosteroids, irradiation, or immunosuppressive agents may be particularly prone to infection. Age, chronic debilitating disease, shock, coma, traumatic injury, or surgical procedures also make a person more susceptible.

TRANSMISSION

Microorganisms are transmitted by various routes, and the same microorganism may be transmitted by more than one route. For example, varicella-zoster virus can spread either by the airborne route, eg, droplet nuclei or by direct contact. The differences in infectivity and in the mode of transmission of the various agents form the basis for the differences in isolation precautions that are recommended in this guideline.

There are 4 main routes of transmission—contact, vehicle, airborne, and vectorborne.

1. Contact transmission, the most important and frequent means of transmission of nosocomial infections, can be divided into 3 subgroups: direct contact, indirect contact, and droplet contact.
   a. Direct contact—This involves direct physical transfer between a susceptible host and an infected or colonized person, such as occurs when hospital personnel turn patients, give baths, change dressings, or perform other procedures requiring direct personal contact. Direct contact can also occur between 2 patients, 1 serving as the source of infection and the other as a susceptible host.
   b. Indirect contact—This involves personal contact of the susceptible host with a contaminated intermediate object, usually inanimate, such as bed linens, clothing, instruments, and dressings.
   c. Droplet contact—Infectious agents may come in contact with the conjunctivae, nose, or mouth of a susceptible person as a result of coughing, sneezing, or talking by an infected person who has clinical disease or is a carrier of the organism. This is considered "contact" transmission rather than airborne since droplets usually travel no more than about 3 feet.
2. The vehicle route applies in diseases transmitted through these contaminated items:
   a. food, such as in salmonellosis;
   b. water, such as in legionellosis;
   c. drugs, such as in bacteremia resulting from infusion of a contaminated infusion product;
   d. blood, such as in hepatitis B, or non-A, non-B hepatitis.
3. Airborne transmission occurs by dissemination of either droplet nuclei, ie, residue of evaporated droplets that may remain suspended in the air for long periods of time, or dust particles in the air containing the infectious agent. Organisms carried in this manner can be widely dispersed by air currents before being inhaled or deposited on the susceptible host.
4. Vectorborne transmission is of greater concern in tropical countries, eg, with mosquito-transmitted malaria. It is of little significance in hospitals in the United States.

Isolation precautions are designed to prevent the spread of microorganisms among patients, personnel, and visitors. Since agent and host factors are more difficult to control, interruption of the chain of infection in the hospital is directed primarily at transmission. The isolation precautions recommended in this guideline are based on this concept.

Nevertheless, placing a patient on isolation precautions often presents certain disadvantages to both the hospital and the patient. Some isolation precautions may be time-consuming and add to the cost of hospitalization. They may make frequent visits by physicians, nurses, and other personnel inconvenient, and they may make it difficult for hospital personnel to give the prompt and frequent care that is sometimes required. The occasional recommendation of a private room under some circumstances uses valuable space that might otherwise accommodate several patients. Moreover, forced solitude deprives the patient of normal social relationships and may be psychologically injurious, especially for children. In an attempt to balance the disadvantages of placing a patient on isolation precautions against the various hazards posed by transmissible infections, "degrees of isolation" have been designated.

In general, it is safer to "over-isolate" than to "under-isolate," particularly when the diagnosis is uncertain and several diseases are seriously being considered. For the patient who appears to have a disease requiring isolation precautions, it is important to institute appropriate isolation precautions immediately rather than wait for confirmation of the diagnosis. Furthermore, certain general precautions may be required even though the patient does not fully meet the criteria for specific isolation precautions. For example, patients with bacteriuria and indwelling urinary catheters are known to serve as reservoirs of infection for roommates who also have indwelling urinary catheters. Passive carriage on the hands of personnel who provide urinary catheter care transmits these infections. Thus, noninfected patients with catheters should not, *where practical*, share rooms with catheterized patients who have bacteriuria.

Isolation precautions also may have to be modified for a patient who needs constant care or whose clinical condition may require emergency intervention such as those in intensive care units or nurseries. When such modifications are made, it is essential that the risk to other patients or hospital personnel of acquiring nosocomial infection be minimized.

RESPONSIBILITY FOR CARRYING OUT PRECAUTIONS

The hospital is responsible for ensuring that patients are placed on appropriate isolation precautions. Each hospital should designate clearly, as a matter of policy, the personnel responsible for placing a patient on isolation precautions and the personnel who have the ultimate authority to make decisions regarding isolation precautions when conflicts arise.

All personnel—physicians, nurses, technicians, students, and others—are responsible for complying with isolation precautions and for tactfully calling observed infractions to the attention of offenders. Physicians should observe the proper isolation precautions at all times; they must teach by example. The responsibilities of hospital personnel for carrying out isolation precautions cannot be effectively dictated but must arise from a personal sense of responsibility.

Patients also have a responsibility for complying with isolation precautions. The appropriate measures should be explained to the patient by physicians and nurses. An important general patient responsibility is handwashing after touching infective material and potentially contaminated articles.

Infractions of the isolation protocol by some are sufficient to negate the conscientious efforts of others. The maxim, ''The chain is no stronger than its weakest link,'' is certainly true.

TECHNIQUES

Many techniques and recommendations for isolation precautions are appropriate not only for patients with known or suspected infection, but also for routine patient care. It is appropriate to use gowns for patient care when soiling with feces is likely, whether or not the patient is infected with an enteric pathogen. Caution when handling hypodermic needles and syringes is appropriate at all times.

HANDWASHING

Handwashing is the single most important means of preventing the spread of infection. Personnel should always wash their hands, even when gloves are used, after taking care of an infected patient or one who is colonized with microorganisms of special clinical or epidemiologic significance, eg, multiply-resistant bacteria. In addition, personnel should wash their hands after touching excretions, eg, feces, urine, or material soiled with them, or secretions, eg, from wounds, skin infections, etc., before touching any patient again. Hands should also be washed before performing invasive procedures, touching wounds, or touching patients who are particularly susceptible to infection. Hands should be washed between all patient contacts in intensive care units and newborn nurseries.

When taking care of patients infected, or colonized, with virulent or epidemiologically important microorganisms, personnel should consider using antiseptics for handwashing rather than soap and water, especially in intensive care units. Antiseptics will inhibit or kill many microorganisms that may not be completely removed by normal handwashing; antiseptics that have a residual effect will continue to suppress microbial growth well after handwashing. Such antiseptics should not be used as a substitute for adequate handwashing, however.

PRIVATE ROOM

In general, a private room can reduce the possibility of transmission of infectious agents in two ways. First, it separates infected or colonized patients from susceptible patients and thus lessens the chance for transmission by any route. Second, it may act as a reminder for personnel to wash their hands before leaving the room and contacting other patients, especially if a sink is available at the doorway. Nevertheless, a private room is not necessary to prevent the spread of many infections.

A private room is indicated for patients with infections that are highly infectious or are caused by microorganisms that are likely to be virulent when transmitted. A private room is also indicated if patient hygiene is poor, eg, if a patient does not wash hands after touching infective material (feces and purulent drainage or secretions), contaminates the environment, or shares contaminated articles. Such patients may include infants, children, and patients who have altered mental status. A private room may also be indicated for patients colonized with microorganisms of special clinical or epidemiologic significance, eg, multiply-resistant bacteria. Finally, a private room may be indicated for patients whose blood is infective, eg, hepatitis B, if profuse bleeding is likely to cause environmental contamination.

In addition to handwashing facilities, a private room should contain bathing and toilet facilities if the room is used for patients requiring isolation precautions. Toilet facilities obviate the need for portable commodes or special precautions for transporting commodes, bedpans, and urinals. An anteroom between the room and the hall, especially for rooms housing patients with highly infectious diseases spread by airborne transmission, will help maintain isolation precautions by reducing the possibility of airborne spread of infectious agents from the room into the corridor whenever the door of the room is opened. Anterooms also provide storage space for supplies, such as gowns, gloves, and masks.

For a few infections, a private room with special ventilation is required. Special ventilation results in negative air pressure in the room in relation to the anteroom or hall, when the room door is closed. The ventilation air, which should generally result in 6 air changes per hour, preferably should be discharged outdoors away from intake vents or receive high efficiency filtration before being recirculated to other rooms.

ROOMMATES FOR PATIENTS ON ISOLATION PRECAUTIONS

If infected or colonized patients are not placed in private rooms, they should be placed with appropriate roommates. Generally, infected patients should not share a room with a patient who is likely to become infected, or if consequences of infection are likely to be severe.

When an infected patient shares a room with non-infected patients, it is assumed that patients and personnel will take measures to prevent the spread of infection. For example, a patient whose fecal material is infective may be in a room with others as long as that patient is cooperative, washes hands carefully, and does not have severe diarrhea or fecal incontinence that will cause either roommates, or objects used by them to become contaminated. Likewise, personnel need to wear gloves and wash hands when indicated and ensure that contaminated articles are discarded or returned for decontamination and reprocessing. When these conditions cannot be met, a private room is advisable.

In general, patients infected by the same microorganism may share a room. Also, infants and young children with the same respiratory clinical syndrome, eg, croup, may share a room. Such grouping, or cohorting, of patients is especially useful during outbreaks when there is a shortage of private rooms.

MASKS

In general, masks are recommended to prevent transmission of infectious agents through the air. Masks protect the wearer from inhaling:

1. large-particle aerosols (droplets) that are transmitted by close contact and generally travel only short distances (about 3 feet) and
2. small-particle aerosols (droplet nuclei) that remain suspended in the air and thus travel longer distances.

Masks might also prevent transmission of some infections that are spread by direct contact with mucous membranes, because masks may discourage personnel from touching the mucous membranes of their eyes, nose, and mouth until after they have washed their hands and removed the mask. The high efficiency disposable masks are more effective than cotton gauze or paper tissue masks in preventing airborne and droplet spread.

If the infection is transmitted by large-particle aerosols (droplets), we recommend masks only for those close to the patient. If the infection is transmitted over longer distances by air, we recommend masks for all persons entering the room. When masks are indicated, they should be used only once—masks become ineffective when moist—and discarded in an appropriate receptacle; masks should not be lowered around the neck and reused. All masks should cover both the nose and the mouth.

GOWNS

In general, gowns are recommended to prevent soiling of clothing when taking care of patients, but are not necessary for most patient care because such soiling is not likely. However, gowns are indicated when taking care of patients on isolation precautions if clothes are likely to be soiled with infective secretions or excretions, eg, when changing the bed of an incontinent patient who has infectious diarrhea or when holding an infant who has a respiratory infection. Furthermore, gowns are indicated, even when gross soiling is not anticipated, for all persons entering the room of patients who have infections that if transmitted in hospitals frequently cause serious illness, eg, varicella (chickenpox) or disseminated zoster. When gowns are indicated, they should be worn only once and then discarded in an appropriate receptacle. Clean, freshly laundered or disposable gowns may be worn in most circumstances. In some instances, as with extensive burns or extensive wounds, sterile gowns may be worn when changing dressings.

GLOVES

In general, there are 3 distinct reasons for wearing gloves. First, gloves reduce the possibility that personnel will become infected with microorganisms that are infecting patients; for example, gloves should prevent personnel from developing herpetic whitlow after giving oral care or suctioning a patient with oral herpes simplex infections. Second, gloves reduce the likelihood that personnel will transmit their own endogenous microbial flora to patients; for example, sterile gloves are used for this reason when personnel perform operations or touch open surgical wounds. Third, gloves reduce the possibility that personnel will become transiently colonized with microorganisms that can be transmitted to other patients. Under most conditions, such transient colonization can be eliminated by handwashing. Thus, in hospitals where handwashing is performed carefully and appropriately by all personnel, gloves are theoretically not necessary to prevent transient colonization of personnel and subsequent transmission by them to others. However, since handwashing practices are thought to be inadequate in most hospitals, gloves appear to be a practical means of preventing transient hand colonization and spread of some infections. Therefore, for many diseases or conditions listed in this guideline, wearing gloves is indicated for touching the excretions, secretions, blood, or body fluids that are listed as infective material. Gloves may not be needed if "no touch" technique (not touching infective materials with hands) can be used.

When gloves are indicated, disposable single-use gloves, ie, sterile or nonsterile, depending on the purpose for use, should be worn. Used gloves should be discarded into an appropriate receptacle. After direct contact with a patient's excretions or secretions, when taking care of that patient, gloves should be changed if care of that patient has not been completed.

DISPOSAL OF ARTICLES

Used articles may need to be enclosed in an impervious bag before they are removed from the room or cubicle of a patient on isolation precautions. Such bagging is intended to prevent inadvertent exposures of personnel to articles contaminated with infective material and prevent contamination of the environment. Most articles do not need to be bagged unless they are contaminated, or likely to be contaminated, with infective material. A single bag is probably adequate if the bag is impervious and sturdy, ie, not easily penetrated, and if the article can be placed in the bag without contaminating the outside of the bag; otherwise, double bagging should be used. Bags should be labeled or be a particular color designated solely for contaminated articles or infectious wastes.

DISPOSAL OF EQUIPMENT

A variety of disposable patient care equipment is available and should be considered for patients on isolation precautions. Use of these disposable articles reduces the possibility that equipment will serve as a fomite, but they must be disposed of safely and adequately. Equipment that is contaminated, or likely to be contaminated, with infective material should be bagged, labeled, and disposed of in accordance with the hospital's policy for disposal of infectious wastes. Local regulations may call for incineration or disposal in an authorized sanitary landfill without the bag's being opened. No special precautions are indicated for disposable patient care equipment that is not contaminated, or likely to be contaminated, with infective material.

REUSABLE EQUIPMENT

Ideally, such equipment should be returned to a central processing area for decontamination and reprocessing by trained personnel. When contaminated with infective material, equipment should be bagged and labeled before being removed from the patient's room or cubicle and remain bagged until decontaminated or sterilized. Special procedure trays should be separated into component parts and handled appropriately (some components can be discarded; others may need to be sent to the laundry or central services for reprocessing).

NEEDLES AND SYRINGES

In general, personnel should use caution when handling all used needles and syringes because it is usually not known which patient's blood is contaminated with hepatitis virus or other microorganisms. To prevent needle-stick injuries, used needles should not be recapped; they should be placed in a prominently labeled, puncture-resistant container designated specifically for this purpose. Needles should not be purposely bent or broken by hand, because accidental needle puncture may occur. When some needle-cutting devices are used, blood may spatter onto environmental surfaces; however, currently no data are available from controlled studies examining the effect, if any, of these devices on the incidence of needle-transmissible infections. If the patient's blood is infective, disposable syringes and needles are preferred. If reusable syringes are used, they should be bagged and returned for decontamination and reprocessing.

SPHYGMOMANOMETER AND STETHOSCOPE

No special precautions are indicated unless the equipment is contaminated, or likely to be contaminated, with infective material. If contaminated, the equipment should be disinfected in the manner appropriate to the object and to the etiologic agent that necessitated isolation precautions.

THERMOMETERS

Thermometers from patients on isolation precautions should be sterilized or receive high-level disinfection before being used by another patient.

LINEN

In general, soiled linen should be handled as little as possible and with a minimum of agitation to prevent gross microbial contamination of the air and of persons handling the linen. Soiled linen from patients on isolation precautions should be put in a laundry bag in the patient's room or cubicle. The bag should be labeled or be a particular color, eg, red, specifically designated for such linen so that whoever receives the linen knows to take the necessary precautions. Linens will require less handling if the bag is hot-water soluble because such bags can be placed directly into the washing machine. However, a hot-water soluble bag may need to be double bagged because they are generally easily punctured or torn or may dissolve when wet. Linen from patients on isolation precautions should not be sorted before being laundered. If mattresses and pillows are covered with impervious plastic, they can be cleaned by wiping with a disinfectant-detergent.

DISHES

No special precautions are necessary for dishes unless they are visibly contaminated with infective material, eg, with blood, drainage, or secretions. Disposable dishes contaminated with infective material can be handled as disposable patient care equipment. Reusable dishes, utensils, and trays contaminated with infective material should be bagged and labeled before being returned to the food service department. Food service personnel who handle these dishes should wear gloves, and they should wash their hands before handling clean dishes or food.

DRINKING WATER

No special precautions are indicated for drinking water. Containers used to hold water for patients on isolation precautions and glasses should be handled as dishes.

DRESSINGS AND TISSUES

All dressings, paper tissues, and other disposable items soiled with infective material, eg, respiratory, oral, or wound secretions, should be bagged, labeled, and disposed of in accordance with the hospital's policy for disposal of infectious wastes. Local regulations may call for incineration or disposal in an authorized sanitary landfill without being opened.

URINE AND FECES

Urine and feces from patients on isolation precautions can be flushed down the toilet if the hospital uses a municipal or other safe sewage treatment system. A urinal or bedpan from a patient on isolation precautions should be cleaned and disinfected or sterilized before being used by another patient.

LABORATORY SPECIMENS

In general, each specimen should be put in a well-constructed container with a secure lid to prevent leaking during transport. Care should be taken when collecting specimens to avoid contamination of the outside of the container. If the outside of the container is visibly contaminated, it should be cleaned, disinfected, or placed in an impervious bag. Specimens from patients on isolation precautions may need to be placed in an impervious bag and labeled before being removed from the room or cubicle; bagging is intended to prevent inadvertent exposures of laboratory or transport personnel to infective material and prevent contamination of the environment. Specimens from patients on isolation precautions may need to be bagged before being sent to the laboratory. This will depend on the kind of specimen and container, the procedures for collecting specimens, and the methods for transporting and receiving specimens in the hospital laboratory.

PATIENT'S CHART

The chart should not be allowed to come into contact with infective material or objects that may be contaminated with infective material.

VISITORS

Visitors should talk with a nurse before entering the room or cubicle of a patient on isolation precautions and, if indicated, should be instructed in the appropriate use of gown, mask, gloves, or other special precautions.

TRANSPORTING PATIENTS

Patients infected with virulent or epidemiologically important microorganisms should leave their room only for essential purposes. Appropriate barriers, eg, masks, impervious dressings, etc., to prevent transmission should be used by the patient and transport personnel. Personnel in the area to which the patient is to be taken should be notified of the impending arrival of the patient and of precautions to be used to prevent transmission of infection. Patients should be alerted to the potential spread of their disease and informed as to how they can assist in maintaining a barrier against transmission of their infection to others.

CLOTHING

Clothing soiled with infective material should be bagged before being sent home or to the hospital laundry; it should be washed with a detergent and, if possible, hot water and bleach.

BOOKS, MAGAZINES, PERSONAL ARTICLES

In general, any of these articles visibly soiled with infective material should be disinfected or destroyed. A child with an infection that may be spread by fomites or by contact transmission should not share toys with other children.

ROUTINE CLEANING

The same routine daily cleaning procedures used in other hospital rooms should be used to clean rooms or cubicles of patients on isolation precautions. Cleaning equipment used in rooms of patients whose infection requires a private room should be disinfected before being used in other patient rooms. For example, dirty water should be discarded, wiping cloths and mop heads should be laundered and thoroughly dried, and buckets should be disinfected before being refilled. If cleaning cloths and mop heads are contaminated with infective material or blood, they should be bagged and labeled before being sent to the laundry.

TERMINAL CLEANING

When isolation precautions have been discontinued, the remaining infection control responsibilities relate to the inanimate environment. Therefore, certain epidemiologic aspects of environmental transmission should be kept in mind by personnel involved with terminal cleaning, ie, cleaning after the patient has been taken off isolation precautions or has ceased to be a source of infection. Although microorganisms may be present on walls, floors, and table tops in rooms used for patients on isolation precautions, these environmental surfaces, unless visibly contaminated, are rarely associated with transmission of infections to others. In contrast, microorganisms on contaminated patient care equipment are frequently associated with transmission of infections to other patients when such equipment is not appropriately decontaminated and reprocessed. Therefore, terminal cleaning should primarily be directed toward those items that have been in direct contact with the patient or in contact with the patient's infective material, ie, excretions, secretions, blood, or body fluids. Disinfectant-detergent solution used during terminal cleaning should be freshly prepared. Terminal cleaning of rooms, or cubicles, consists of the following:

1. Generally, housekeeping personnel should use the same precautions to protect themselves during terminal cleaning that they would use if the patient were still in the room. However, masks are not needed if they had been indicated previously only for direct or close patient contact.
2. All nondisposable receptacles, ie, drainage bottles, urinals, bedpans, flowmeter jars, thermometer holders, etc., should be returned for decontamination and reprocessing. Articles that are contaminated, or likely to be contaminated, with infective material should be bagged and labeled before being sent for decontamination and reprocessing.
3. All disposable items should be discarded. Articles that are contaminated, or likely to be contaminated, with infective material should be bagged, labeled, and disposed of in accordance with the hospital's policy on disposal of infectious wastes. Local regulations may call for the bag's incineration or disposal in an authorized sanitary landfill without being opened. No special precautions are indicated for disposal of items that are not contaminated, or not likely to be contaminated, with infective material.

4. All equipment that is not sent to central services or discarded should be cleaned with a disinfectant-detergent solution.

5. All horizontal surfaces of furniture and mattress covers should be cleaned with a disinfectant-detergent solution.

6. All floors should be wet-vacuumed or mopped with a disinfectant-detergent solution.

7. Routine washing of walls, blinds, and curtains is not indicated; however, these should be washed if they are visibly soiled. Cubicle curtains should be changed if visibly soiled.

8. Disinfectant fogging is an unsatisfactory method of decontaminating air and surfaces and thus should not be used.

9. Airing a room from which a patient has been discharged is not an effective terminal disinfection procedure and is not necessary.

10. The State Health Department and the CDC, Hospital Infections Program, should be consulted about cleaning the room of a patient who has suspected smallpox, Lassa fever, Ebola fever, or other hemorrhagic fevers, ie, Marburg disease.

POST-MORTEM HANDLING OF BODIES

Generally, personnel should use the same precautions to protect themselves during postmortem handling of bodies that they would use if the patient were still alive. However, masks are usually not necessary unless aerosols are expected to be generated. Autopsy personnel should be notified about the patient's disease status so that appropriate precautions can be maintained during and after autopsy. State or local regulations may call for additional special precautions for postmortem handling of bodies.

MISCELLANEOUS

1. Isolation carts—Some institutions use pre-stocked isolation carts that contain equipment and supplies for isolation precautions. These can be wheeled to the general area where needed but should be placed in a clean area. Carts should be kept adequately stocked with all necessary supplies.

2. Admission—If a susceptible person has been exposed recently to an infectious disease requiring isolation precautions, the physician should postpone elective admission or prescribe appropriate isolation precautions for a nonelective admission. This situation is most likely to occur with children or young adults.

3. Prophylaxis and immunization—When used appropriately, prophylactic antimicrobials and active or passive immunization may prevent or ameliorate the course of infections to which patients or personnel have been exposed. These measures should be considered as adjuncts to isolation precautions in preventing the spread of disease.

ALTERNATIVE SYSTEMS FOR ISOLATION PRECAUTIONS

SYSTEM A—CATEGORY SPECIFIC

Category-specific isolation precautions is 1 of 2 isolation systems. Isolation categories are derived by grouping diseases for which similar isolation precautions are indicated. For diseases to be grouped into isolation categories, more isolation precautions must be required for some diseases than only those necessary to prevent transmission of those diseases. Such overuse of isolation precautions may be avoided by using the System B—Disease-Specific method. Category-specific isolation precautions, however, are easier to teach and administer.

Seven isolation categories are used:

1. Strict Isolation; yellow card
2. Contact Isolation; orange card
3. Respiratory Isolation; blue card
4. Tuberculosis (AFB) Isolation; grey card
5. Enteric Precautions; brown card
6. Drainage/Secretion Precautions; green card
7. Blood/Body Fluid Precautions violet card

Strict Isolation ''Strict Isolation'' is an isolation category designed to prevent transmission of highly contagious or virulent infections that may be spread by both air and contact.

Specifications for Strict Isolation

1. Private room is indicated; door should be kept closed. In general, patients infected with the same organism may share a room.
2. Masks are indicated for all persons entering the room.
3. Gowns are indicated for all persons entering the room.
4. Gloves are indicated for all persons entering the room.
5. Hands must be washed after touching the patient or potentially contaminated articles and before taking care of another patient.
6. Articles contaminated with infective material should be discarded or bagged and labeled before being sent for decontamination and reprocessing.

Diseases Requiring Strict Isolation

Diphtheria, pharyngeal
Lassa fever and other viral hemorrhagic fevers, ie, Marburg virus disease*
Plague, pneumonic
Smallpox*
Varicella (chickenpox)
Zoster, localized in immunocompromised patient or disseminated

Contact Isolation ''Contact Isolation'' is designed to prevent transmission of highly transmissible or epidemiologically important infections, or colonization, that do not warrant Strict Isolation. All diseases or conditions included in this category are spread primarily by close or direct contact. Thus, masks, gowns, and gloves are recommended for anyone in close or direct contact with any patient who has an infection, or colonization, that is included in this category. For individual diseases or conditions, however, 1 or more of these 3 barriers may not be indicated. For example, masks and gloves are not generally indicated for care of infants and young children with acute viral respiratory infections, gowns are not generally indicated for gonococcal conjunctivitis in newborns, and masks are not generally indicated for care of patients infected with multiply-resistant microorganisms, except those with pneumonia. Therefore, some degree of ''over-isolation'' may occur in this category.

---

*A private room with special ventilation is indicated.

Specifications for Contact Isolation

1. Private room is indicated. In general, patients infected with the same organism may share a room. During outbreaks, infants and young children with the same respiratory clinical syndrome may share a room.
2. Masks are indicated for those who come close to the patient.
3. Gowns are indicated if soiling is likely.
4. Gloves are indicated for touching infective material.
5. Hands must be washed after touching the patient or potentially contaminated articles and before taking care of another patient.
6. Articles contaminated with infective material should be discarded or bagged and labeled before being sent for decontamination and re-processing.

Diseases or Conditions Requiring Contact Isolation

Acute respiratory infections in infants and young children, including croup, colds, bronchitis, and bronchiolitis caused by respiratory syncytial virus, adenovirus, coronavirus, influenza viruses, parainfluenza viruses, and rhinovirus

Conjunctivitis, gonococcal, in newborns

Diphtheria, cutaneous

Endometritis, group A *Streptococcus*

Furunculosis, staphylococcal, in newborns

Herpes simplex, disseminated, severe primary or neonatal

Impetigo

Influenza, in infants and young children

Multiply-resistant bacteria, infection or colonization (any site) with any of the following:

1. Gram-negative bacilli resistant to all aminoglycosides that are tested. (In general, such organisms should be resistant to gentamicin, tobramycin, and amikacin for these special precautions to be indicated.)
2. *Staphylococcus aureus* resistant to methicillin (or nafcillin or oxacillin if they are used instead of methicillin for testing)
3. *Pneumococcus* resistant to penicillin
4. *Haemophilus influenzae* resistant to ampicillin (beta-lactamase positive) and chloramphenicol
5. Other resistant bacteria may be included if they are judged by the infection control team to be of special clinical and epidemiologic significance.

Pediculosis

Pharyngitis, infectious, in infants and young children

Pneumonia, viral, in infants and young children

Pneumonia, *Staphylococcus aureus* or group A *Streptococcus*

Rabies

Rubella, congenital and other

Scabies

Scalded skin syndrome, staphylococcal (Ritter's disease)

Skin, wound, or burn infection, major (draining and not covered by dressing or dressing does not adequately contain the purulent material) including those infected with *Staphylococcus aureus* or group A *Streptococcus*

Vaccinia (generalized and progressive eczema vaccinatum)

Respiratory Isolation "Respiratory Isolation" is designed to prevent transmission of infectious diseases primarily over short distances through the air (droplet transmission). Direct and indirect contact transmission occurs with some infections in this isolation category but is infrequent.

Specifications for Respiratory Isolation

1. Private room is indicated. In general, patients infected with the same organism may share a room.
2. Masks are indicated for those who come close to the patient.
3. Gowns are not indicated.
4. Gloves are not indicated.
5. Hands must be washed after touching the patient or potentially contaminated articles and before taking care of another patient.
6. Articles contaminated with infective material should be discarded or bagged and labeled before being sent for decontamination and reprocessing.

Diseases Requiring Respiratory Isolation

Epiglottitis, *Haemophilus influenzae*
Erythema infectiosum
Measles
Meningitis
  Haemophilus influenzae, known or suspected
  Meningococcal, known or suspected
Meningococcal pneumonia
Meningococcemia
Mumps
Pertussis (whooping cough)
Pneumonia, *Haemophilus influenzae,* in children (any age)

Tuberculosis (AFB) Isolation ''Tuberculosis (AFB) Isolation'' is an isolation category for patients with pulmonary TB who have a positive sputum smear or a chest X-ray that strongly suggests current (active) TB. Laryngeal TB is also included in this isolation category. In general, infants and young children with pulmonary TB do not require isolation precautions because they rarely cough, and their bronchial secretions contain few AFB, compared with adults with pulmonary TB. On the instruction card, this category is called AFB (for acid-fast bacilli) Isolation to protect the patient's privacy.

Specifications for Tuberculosis Isolation (AFB Isolation)

1. Private room with special ventilation is indicated; door should be kept closed. In general, patients infected with the same organism may share a room.
2. Masks are indicated only if the patient is coughing and does not reliably cover mouth.
3. Gowns are indicated only if needed to prevent gross contamination of clothing.
4. Gloves are not indicated.
5. Hands must be washed after touching the patient or potentially contaminated articles and before taking care of another patient.
6. Articles are rarely involved in transmission of TB. However, articles should be thoroughly cleaned and disinfected, or discarded.

Enteric Precautions ''Enteric Precautions'' are designed to prevent infections that are transmitted by direct or indirect contact with feces. Hepatitis A is included in this category because it is spread through feces, although the disease is much less likely to be transmitted after the onset of jaundice. Most infections in this category primarily cause gastrointestinal symptoms, but some do not. For example, feces from patients infected with ''poliovirus'' and coxsackieviruses are infective, but these infections do not usually cause prominent gastrointestinal symptoms.

Specifications for Enteric Precautions

1. Private room is indicated if patient hygiene is poor. A patient with poor hygiene does not wash hands after touching infective material, contaminates the environment with infective material, or shares contaminated articles with other patients. In general, patients infected with the same organism may share a room.
2. Masks are not indicated.
3. Gowns are indicated if soiling is likely.
4. Gloves are indicated if touching infective material.
5. Hands must be washed after touching the patient or potentially contaminated articles and before taking care of another patient.
6. Articles contaminated with infective material should be discarded or bagged and labeled before being sent for decontamination and re-processing.

Diseases Requiring Enteric Precautions

Amebic dysentery
Cholera
Coxsackievirus disease
Diarrhea, acute illness with suspected infectious etiology
Echovirus disease
Encephalitis (unless known not to be caused by enteroviruses)
Enterocolitis caused by *Clostridium difficile* or *Staphylococcus aureus*
Enteroviral infection
Gastroenteritis caused by
  Campylobacter species
  Cryptosporidium species
  Dientameoba fragilis
  Escherichia coli (enterotoxic, enteropathogenic, or enteroinvasive)
  Giardia lamblia
  Salmonella species
  Shigella species
  Vibrio parahaemolyticus
  Viruses—including Norwalk agent and rotavirus
  Yersinia enterocolitica
  Unknown etiology but presumed to be an infectious agent
Hand, foot, and mouth disease
Hepatitis, viral, type A
Herpangina
Meningitis, viral (unless known not to be caused by enteroviruses)
Necrotizing enterocolitis
Pleurodynia
Poliomyelitis
Typhoid fever (*Salmonella typhi*)
Viral pericarditis, myocarditis, or meningitis (unless known not to be caused by enteroviruses).

Drainage/Secretion Precautions "Drainage/Secretion Precautions" are designed to prevent infections that are transmitted by direct or indirect contact with purulent material or drainage from an infected body site. This newly created isolation category includes many infections formerly included in Wound and Skin Precautions, Discharge (lesion), and Secretion (oral) Precautions, which have been discontinued. Infectious diseases included in this category are those that result in the production of infective purulent material, drainage, or secretions, unless the disease is included in another isolation category that requires more rigorous precautions. For example, minor or limited skin, wound, or burn infections are included in this category, but major skin, wound, or burn infections are included in Contact Isolation.

Specifications for Drainage/Secretion Precautions

1. Private room is not indicated.
2. Masks are not indicated.
3. Gowns are indicated if soiling is likely.
4. Gloves are indicated for touching infective material.
5. Hands must be washed after touching the patient or potentially contaminated articles and before taking care of another patient.
6. Articles contaminated with infective material should be discarded or bagged and labeled before being sent for decontamination and re-processing.

Diseases Requiring Drainage/Secretion Precautions

The following infections are examples of those included in this category provided they are *not* (1) caused by multiply-resistant microorganisms, (2) major (draining and not covered by a dressing or dressing does not adequately contain the drainage) skin, wound, or burn infections, including those caused by *Staphylococcus aureus* or group A *Streptococcus,* or (3) gonococcal eye infections in newborns. See Contact Isolation if the infection is 1 of these 3.

Abscess, minor or limited
Burn infection, minor or limited
Conjunctivitis
Decubitus ulcer, infected, minor or limited
Skin infection, minor or limited
Wound infection, minor or limited

Blood/Body Fluid Precautions ''Blood/Body Fluid Precautions'' are designed to prevent infections that are transmitted by direct or indirect contact with infective blood or body fluids. Infectious diseases included in this category are those that result in the production of infective blood or body fluids, unless the disease is included in another isolation category that requires more rigorous precautions, for example, Strict Isolation. For some diseases included in this category, such as malaria, only blood is infective; for other diseases, such as hepatitis B (including antigen carriers), blood and body fluids (saliva, semen, etc.) are infective.

Specifications for Blood/Body Fluid Precautions

1. Private room is indicated if patient hygiene is poor. A patient with poor hygiene does not wash hands after touching infective material, contaminates the environment with infective material, or shares contaminated articles with other patients. In general, patients infected with the same organism may share a room.
2. Masks are not indicated.
3. Gowns are indicated if soiling of clothing with blood or body fluids is likely.
4. Gloves are indicated for touching blood or body fluids.
5. Hands must be washed immediately if they are potentially contaminated with blood or body fluids and before taking care of another patient.
6. Articles contaminated with blood or body fluids should be discarded or bagged and labeled before being sent for decontamination and reprocessing.

7. Care should be taken to avoid needle-stick injuries. Used needles should not be recapped or bent; they should be placed in a prominently labeled, puncture-resistant container designated specifically for such disposal.
8. Blood spills should be cleaned up promptly with a solution of 5.25% sodium hypochlorite diluted 1:10 with water.

Diseases Requiring Blood/Body Fluid Precautions

Acquired immunodeficiency syndrome (AIDS)
Arthropodborne viral fevers, eg, dengue, yellow fever, and Colorado tick fever
Babesiosis
Creutzfeldt-Jakob disease
Hepatitis B (including HBsAg antigen carrier)
Hepatitis, non-A, non-B
Leptospirosis
Malaria
Rat-bite fever
Relapsing fever
Syphilis, primary and secondary with skin and mucous membrane lesions

SYSTEM B—DISEASE SPECIFIC

Disease-specific isolation precautions is 1 of 2 isolation systems. Either the category-specific (System A) or the disease-specific (System B) isolation system should be chosen by the institution. Elements of both cannot be combined easily. With disease-specific isolation precautions, each infectious disease is considered individually. Therefore, only those precautions specific to the identified disease need to be implemented. The advantage of the disease-specific isolation precautions system is a savings of supplies and expense. Excessive donning of masks, gowns, and gloves is avoided, saving time and inconvenience. This inconvenience may also cause a lack of proper adherence to necessary precautions.

Isolation precautions are often most important during the early stages of a patient's treatment, prior to establishing a definitive diagnosis and implementing a specific treatment protocol. In these cases, category-specific precautions, which are more general, and thus offer a wider spectrum of protection, may be more practical and easier to implement.

Because the risk of transmission, and the subsequent consequences of infection are greater in infants and young children than for adults, more stringent isolation precautions for infants and young children are recommended.

A list of the instruction cards used to denote isolation precaution conditions by isolation category and color designation are listed on page 89.
When isolation precautions are imposed, information required to complete the cards should be filled in completely and legibly. Cards are conspicuously posted in the immediate area of the patient. Duplicates may be posted on the front of the patient's chart.

This information, including complete listings for Systems A and B is available in the CDC Guideline for Isolation Precautions in Hospitals (PB85-923401), produced by the Center for Infectious Diseases, CDC. For application in clinical settings, updated information from the CDC, and information specific to the institution, should be sought.

MODIFICATION OF ISOLATION PRECAUTIONS

INTENSIVE CARE

Patients requiring intensive care are usually at higher risk than other patients of becoming colonized or infected with organisms of special clinical or epidemiologic significance. Three reasons are that contacts between these patients and personnel are frequent, the patients are clustered in a confined area, and many of them are unusually susceptible to infection. Moreover, critically ill patients are more likely to have multiple invasive procedures performed on them. Because there is ample opportunity for cross-infection in the Intensive Care Unit (ICU), infection control precautions must be done scrupulously. Frequent in-service training and close supervision to ensure adequate application of infection control and isolation precautions are particularly important for ICU personnel.

Most ICUs pose special problems for applying isolation precautions. Modifications that will neither compromise patient care nor increase the risk of infection to other patients or personnel may be necessary. Isolation precaution that will most often have to be modified is the use of a private room. Ideally, private rooms should be available in ICUs, but some ICUs do not have them or do not use them for patients who are critically ill if frequent and easy accessibility by personnel is crucial. When a private room is not available or is not desirable because of the patient's critical condition, and if airborne transmission is *not* likely, an isolation area can be defined within the ICU by curtains, partitions, or an area marked off on the floor with tape. Instructional cards can be posted to inform personnel and visitors about the isolation precautions in use.

Patients with infections that can cause serious illness, eg, chickenpox, if transmitted in hospitals, should be put in a private room even when the ICU does not have one. Because the risk of these highly contagious or virulent infections to patients and personnel is great, the inconvenience and expense associated with intensive care in a private room outside the ICU must be accepted.

One isolation precaution that should never be modified in intensive care units is frequent and appropriate handwashing. Hands should be washed between patients and may need to be washed several times during the care of a patient so that microorganisms are not transmitted from one site to another on the same patient; eg, from urinary tract to wound. Antiseptics, rather than soap, should be considered for handwashing in intensive care units.

INFANTS AND NEWBORNS

Isolation precautions for newborns and infants may have to be modified from those recommended for adults because:

1. Usually only a small number of private rooms are available for newborns and infants; and
2. During outbreaks, it is frequently necessary to establish cohorts of newborns and infants.

Moreover, a newborn may need to be placed on isolation precautions at delivery because its mother has an infection.

It has often been recommended that infected newborns or those suspected of being infected (regardless of the pathogen and clinical manifestations) should be put in a private room. This recommendation was based on the assumptions that a geographically isolated room was necessary to protect uninfected newborns and that infected newborns would receive closer scrutiny and better care in such a room. Neither of these assumptions is completely correct.

Separate isolation rooms are seldom indicated for newborns with many kinds of infection if the following conditions are met:

1. An adequate number of nursing and medical personnel are on duty and have sufficient time for appropriate handwashing;
2. Sufficient space is available for a 4- to 6-foot aisle or area between newborn stations;
3. An adequate number of sinks for handwashing are available in each nursery room or area; and
4. Continuing instruction is given to personnel about the mode of transmission of infections.

When these criteria are not met, a separate room with handwashing facilities may be indicated.

Another incorrect assumption regarding isolation precautions for newborns and infants is that forced-air incubators can be substituted for private rooms. These incubators may filter the incoming air but not the air discharged into the nursery. Moreover, the surfaces of incubators housing newborns or infants can easily become contaminated with organisms infecting or colonizing the patient, so personnel working with the patient through portholes may have their hands and forearms colonized. Forced-air incubators, therefore, are satisfactory for limited ''protective'' isolation of newborns and infants but should not be relied on as a major means of preventing transmission from infected patients to others.

Isolation precautions for an infected or colonized newborn or infant, or for a newborn of a mother suspected of having an infectious disease can be determined by the specific viral or bacterial pathogen, the clinical manifestations, the source and possible modes of transmission, and the number of colonized or infected newborns or infants. Other factors to be considered include the overall condition of the newborn or infant and the kind of care required, the available space and facilities, the nurse-to-patient ratio, and the size and type of nursery services for newborns and infants.

In addition to applying isolation precautions, cohorts may be established to keep to a minimum the transmission of organisms or infectious diseases among different groups of newborns and infants in large nurseries. A cohort usually consists of all well newborns from the same 24- or 48-hour birth period; these newborns are admitted to and kept in a single nursery room and, ideally, are taken care of by a single group of personnel who do not take care of any other cohort during the same shift. After the newborns in a cohort have been discharged, the room is thoroughly cleaned and prepared to accept the next cohort.

Cohorting is not practical as a routine for small nurseries or in neonatal intensive care units or graded care nurseries. It is useful in these nurseries, however, as a control measure during outbreaks or for managing a group of infants or newborns colonized or infected with an epidemiologically important pathogen. Under these circumstances, having separate rooms for each cohort is ideal, but not mandatory for many kinds of infections if cohorts can be kept separate within a single large room and if personnel are assigned to take care of only those in the cohort.

During outbreaks, newborns or infants with overt infection or colonization and personnel who are carriers, if indicated, should be identified rapidly and placed in cohorts; if rapid identification is not possible, exposed newborns or infants should be placed in a cohort separate from those with disease and from unexposed infants and newborns and new admissions. The success of cohorting depends largely on the willingness and ability of nursing and ancillary personnel to adhere strictly to the cohort system and to meticulously follow patient care practices.

SEVERELY COMPROMISED PATIENTS

Patients with certain diseases, such as cancer or burns, and patients who are receiving certain therapeutic regimens, such as total body irradiation or steroids, are highly susceptible to infection. Such patients are considered to be severely compromised because the basic disease process from which they suffer, or the therapeutic regimen for treatment, makes them more susceptible to the transmission of infection.

The use of "Protective Isolation" does not appear to reduce this risk any more than strong emphasis on appropriate handwashing during patient care. Protective Isolation may fail to reduce the risk of infection because compromised patients are often infected by their own (endogenous) microorganisms or are colonized and infected by microorganisms transmitted by the inadequately washed hands of personnel or by nonsterile items used in routine protective isolation. Such items may include patient care equipment, food, water, and air. Vigorous efforts to exclude all microorganisms by using patient-isolator units, eradicating endogenous flora, and sterilizing food, water, and fomites may prevent or delay onset of some infections; thus, these procedures have been recommended by some for use with very-high-risk patients who have a predictable temporary period of high susceptibility. However, these extraordinary and expensive precautions do not appear warranted for most compromised patients.

In general, compromised patients should be taken care of by using precautions that are no different from routine good patient-care techniques, but for these patients, routine techniques must be emphasized and enforced. All personnel must frequently and appropriately wash their hands before, during, and after patient care. Compromised patients should be kept separate from patients who are infected or have conditions that make infection transmission likely. Private rooms should be used whenever possible.

BURNS

Burn wounds have been classified as major or minor according to several risk factors for burn-associated complications. Only the infectious complications of burns are considered here. Major burn wounds are classified as those that cannot be covered effectively, or whose drainage cannot be contained effectively by use of dressings. The drainage from a minor burn can be covered and contained by dressings.

Most major burn wounds and many minor ones have become infected by the second or third day after the burn occurs. Care of burn patients, therefore, involves efforts to prevent colonization and infection of the wound, and isolation precautions to prevent transmission to other patients. Other important methods of care include use of topical and systemic antimicrobials, vaccines, and general supportive measures. Burn wounds have been grouped under the subheading "skin, wound, or burn infection."

Isolation precautions and infection control techniques for major burn wounds vary among burn centers. These precautions may involve the use of strictly enforced, frequent handwashing, sterile gowns, sterile gloves, and masks. Because it is not possible to "isolate" a major wound by use of dressings, a private room or a special burn center is indicated for such patients.

REFERENCES

1. Favero MS. Chemical disinfection of medical and surgical materials. In: Block SS, ed. *Disinfection, Sterilization, and Preservation.* 3rd ed. Philadelphia: Lea and Febiger; 1983:469–492.
2. Centers for Disease Control. Guideline for Handwashing and Hospital Environmental Control, 1985. PB85-923404. 1985:2.
3. The tentative final monograph for OTC topical antimicrobial products. *Federal Register.* January 1978, 6:43 FR 1210:1211–49T.
4. Lowbury EJL, Lilly HA, Bull JP. Disinfection of hands: Removal of transient organisms. *Br Med J.* 1964; 2:230–233.
5. Sprunt K, Redman W, Leidy G. Antibacterial effectiveness of routine handwashing. *Pediatrics.* 1973; 52:264–271.
6. Ojajarvi J. The importance of soap selection for routine hygiene in hospitals. *J Hyg* (Lond). 1981; 86:275–283.
7. Albert RK, Condie F. Handwashing patterns in medical intensive care units. *N Engl J Med.* 1981; 304:1465–1466.
8. Larson E. Compliance with isolation techniques. *Am J Infect Control.* 1983; 11:221–225.
9. Occupational exposure to ethylene oxide. *Federal Register.* June 22, 1984; 29 CFR 1910.
10. Garner JS, Simmons BP. Guideline for isolation precautions in hospitals. *Infect Control.* 1983; 4:245–325.
11. Centers for Disease Control. Viral hemorrhagic fever: initial management of suspected and confirmed cases. *MMWR.* 1983; 32 (Suppl):275–405.
12. Rutala WA, Stiegel MM, Sarubbi FA. Decontamination of laboratory microbiological waste by steam sterilization. *Appl Environ Microbiol.* 1982; 43:1311–1316.
13. Lauer JL, Battles DR, Vesley D. Decontaminating infectious laboratory waste by autoclaving. *Appl Environ Microbiol.* 1982; 44:690–694.
14. Hughes HG. Chutes in hospitals. *J Can Hosp Assn.* 1964; 41:56–57.
15. Walter WG, Schillinger JE. Bacterial survival in laundered fabrics. *Appl Environ Microbiol.* 1975; 29:368–373.
16. Christian RR, Manchester JT, Mellor MT. Bacteriological quality of fabrics washed at lower-than-standard temperatures in a hospital laundry facility. *Appl Environ Microbiol.* 1983; 45:591–597.
17. Blaser MJ, Smith PF, Cody HJ, et al. Killing of fabric-associated bacteria in hospital laundry by low-temperature washing. *J Infect Dis.* 1984; 149:48–57.

18. Anderson RL, Mackel DC, Stoler BS, et al. Carpeting in hospitals: an epidemiological evaluation. *J Clin Microbiol*. 1982; 15:408–415.
19. American Academy of Pediatrics, American College of Obstetricians and Gynecologists. Guidelines for perinatal care. Evanston, IL and Washington, D.C. AAP, ACOG, 1983.
20. Wysowski DK, Flynt JW, Goldfield M, et al. Epidemic neonatal hyperbilirubinemia and use of a phenolic disinfectant detergent. *Pediatrics*. 1978; 61:165–170.

5
TURNING AND POSITIONING

INTRODUCTION

Patients are sometimes unable to turn in bed or position themselves properly. Frequent turning or repositioning of a dependent patient prevents the development of pressure sores or skin breakdown. A patient must be repositioned at least every two hours. If a patient has problems such as poor circulation, fragile skin, or decreased sensation, more frequent repositioning may be required. When a patient is repositioned, the skin over the area upon which he was lying should be inspected and observed for color and integrity. If recovery is delayed, the patient should be repositioned more frequently. The first time a patient is placed in a new position, check the patient's skin in 5–10 minutes, and frequently thereafter, to determine tolerance for the position. Redness should resolve before pressure is placed again on that area. Excessive redness indicates potential tissue damage.

When sitting a patient must relieve pressure on the buttocks and sacrum at least every ten minutes. Push-ups using the armrests, leaning first to one side and then to the other, and leaning forward are all ways to relieve pressure in the sitting position.

Proper positioning should make the patient as comfortable as possible and prevent development of deformities and pressure sores, as well as provide the patient access to his environment. To achieve these goals, the patient and environment must be properly handled. When turning and repositioning, the patient must be lifted rather than dragged across the sheets to prevent skin irritation. Wrinkles in the sheets, blankets, and clothes should be avoided as they increase pressure on a small area causing skin irritation. Pillows and rolled blankets or towels are used to support body parts to avoid strain on ligaments, nerves, and muscles.

Pillows can be used to provide relief to bony areas, or areas of skin breakdown. The pillows are placed proximally and distally to the involved area.

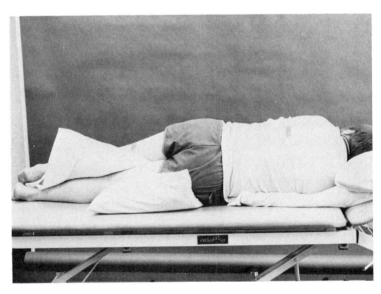

Positioning to bridge the greater trochanter.

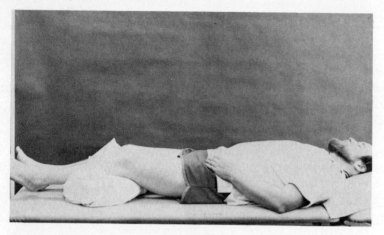

Supine position with pillow under knees.

SUPINE POSITION

In the supine position the shoulders are parallel to the hips with the spine straight. A pillow may be placed under the knees to relieve strain on the lower back.

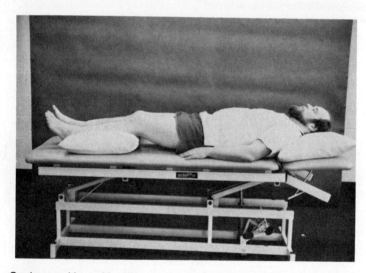

Supine position with pillow under lower legs.

However, this position can lead to decreased hip and knee extension range of motion as a result of prolonged positioning in flexion. A pillow may also be used under the lower leg to relieve pressure on the heels. As an alternative, the feet may be positioned over the end of the bed.

When sheets or blankets are used, they should not be tightly tucked in at the foot of the bed, as that will contribute to decreased ankle dorsiflexion motion. Footboards are occasionally used to maintain the foot in neutral or anatomical position. These are usually ineffective because the patient pushes against the board and the ankle is again in plantarflexion. For some patients stimulation to the sole of the foot causes a reflex that also will result in ankle plantarflexion. Footboards, however, can be used to keep sheets and blankets from forcing the foot into plantarflexion as a result of the weight of the bedding. This is accomplished by placing the bedding over the top edge of the footboard.

TURNING FROM SUPINE TO PRONE

The patient's initial position is supine, and far enough to one side of the bed or mat to allow for a full rolling movement without coming too near the opposite edge. If the patient is to roll to the left, the patient must start at the right of the bed or mat. Complete instructions and explanations should be given to the patient. The patient is moved to the edge of the bed in stages. First the upper trunk,

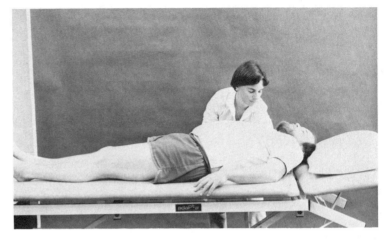

Moving the upper trunk.

then the lower trunk,

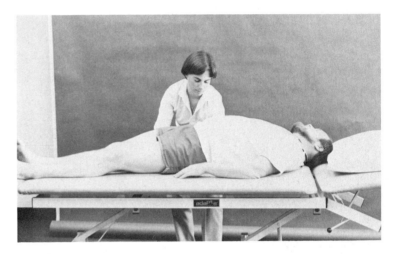

Moving the lower trunk.

and finally the legs are moved.

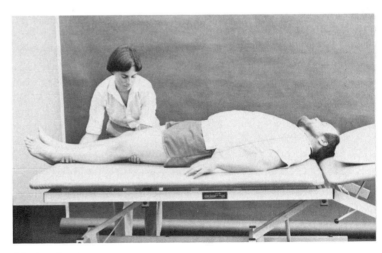

Moving the legs.

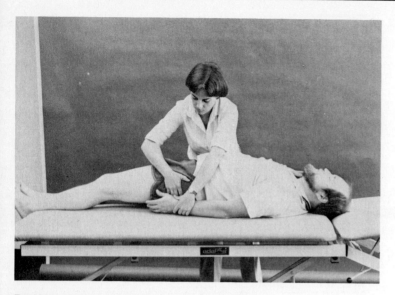

Positioning the upper extremity prior to rolling.

The left upper extremity is adducted so that the hand is placed under the left hip, palm against the hip. The right lower extremity is then crossed over the left lower extremity so that the right ankle is resting on top of the left ankle. The right upper extremity is adducted so that the hand is at the hip, palm against the hip.

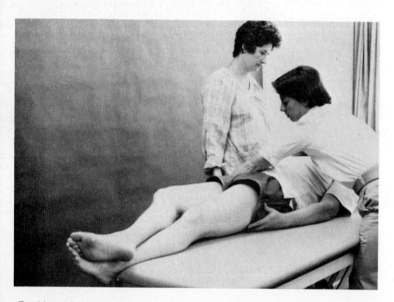

Position of the therapist and assistant at start of turning.

The therapist should be positioned on the side to which the patient is going to be turned. If the bed, or plinth, is narrow, or does not have a guard rail, someone should stand next to the patient to prevent the patient from falling while the therapist moves to the other side of the bed. The second person can assist with positioning pillows and turning the patient. If a pillow is to be placed under the patient for the final positioning, position the pillow so that it will be in the proper position as the patient is rolled.

If the patient has head control, he can assist in turning his head and neck in the direction of the roll as it is initiated. If the patient does not have head and neck control, the therapist must be aware that the patient's face will be subject to some rubbing on the mattress or mat during the roll. When the therapist is ready to initiate the movement, she should indicate that to the patient, give a preparatory count, and then a specific verbal command. The verbal command should be a direct clue to the task.

As the therapist initiates rolling, her hands are on the patient's back. When the patient reaches the half-way point, the patient may finish the roll uncontrolled as a result of the pull of gravity. Therefore, the therapist must rotate her hands as the patient reaches the sidelying position, so that they are on the anterior surface of the patient, controlling the second half of the roll.

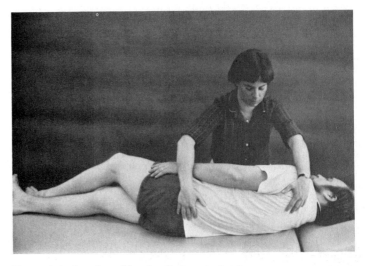

Therapist's hand position for first part of roll.

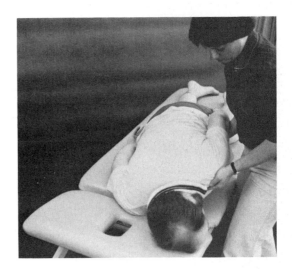

Therapist's hand position for second part of roll.

When the roll is finished, the first body segment to be re-positioned is the head. The head must be placed in a comfortable position facing to one side. There should be no pressure on the eyes, nose, or mouth. After this has been done, the hands should be removed from under the hips. Then the arms should be placed in a position of slight abduction, approximately 20° to 30°. Finally, the feet should be uncrossed if they remain crossed after the roll is finished. They should be placed approximately 6 to 8 inches apart.

PRONE POSITION

In the prone position, the shoulders are parallel to the hips with the spine straight. The head may be turned to either side, or maintained in the midline, with a small pillow or towel under the forehead to increase comfort.

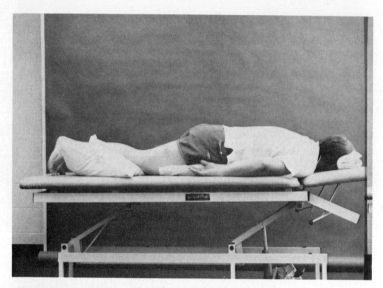

Prone position; arms alongside; pillow under lower legs.

The arms may be positioned alongside the trunk or alongside the head. If the arms are placed alongside the head, the patient should have sensation in the arms, and should be checked frequently for numbness or tingling in the arms. In some patients, circulation to the arms is impaired when the arms are placed alongside the head.

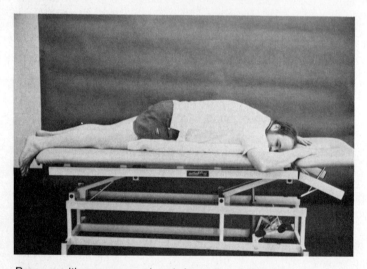

Prone position; arms overhead, feet off end of table.

A pillow under the trunk may be placed lengthwise or crosswise. The lengthwise position may be more comfortable if the patient has limited neck mobility. The crosswise position of the pillow may be more comfortable for a patient with low back pain.

The patient's feet may be positioned over the end of the table. A pillow under the lower legs can also be used to avoid positioning the ankles in plantarflexion. However, the pillow under the lower leg places the knee in slight flexion, and may promote loss of knee extension range of motion.

The crosswise position of the pillow may be used to reduce the lordotic curve of the low back (lumbar region).

TURNING FROM PRONE TO SUPINE

In many respects, rolling from prone to supine is the reverse of rolling from supine to prone. The patient's initial position is prone. The preparatory steps of moving to one side of the bed, and of placement of the patient's hands, remain the same. The crossing of the lower extremities is usually unnecessary.

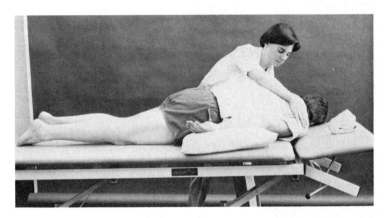

Positioning head and upper trunk for rolling to supine.

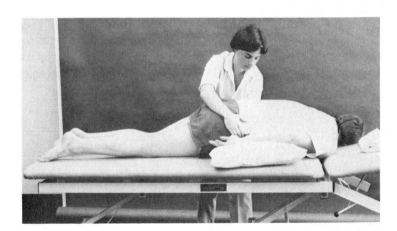

Positioning lower trunk for rolling to supine.

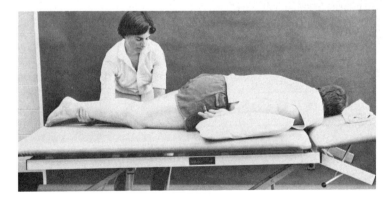

Positioning lower extremities for rolling to supine.

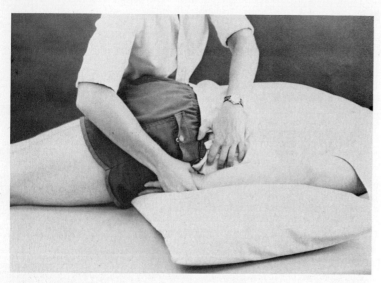

Positioning patient's hand for rolling to supine.

The therapist is again positioned on the side to which the patient will roll. When rolling prone to supine, rubbing of the face on the mattress or mat can be avoided by having the patient start by facing away from the therapist. If the patient has head control, he can assist by looking up and over his shoulder as he is turned towards the therapist. If the plinth is narrow, or the bed lacks a guard rail, an assistant should guard the patient as the therapist moves to the other side of the bed. The assistant can help with positioning of pillows and the patient.

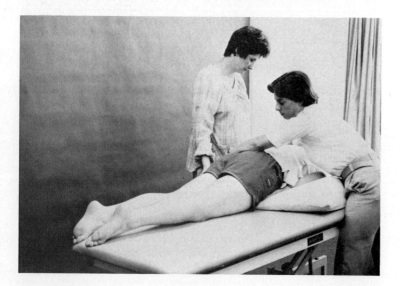

Starting position to roll from prone to supine.

As in rolling from supine to prone, the therapist must control both parts of the rolling motion. Initially, the therapist reaches over the patient and places her hands on the anterior surface. As the patient reaches the sidelying position, the therapist rotates her hands so that they are on the posterior surface of the patient, and can control the second half of the roll.

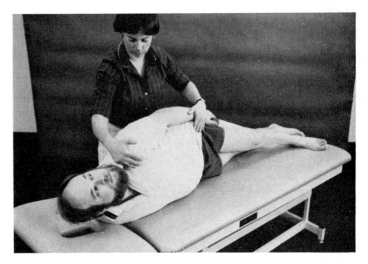

Therapist's hand position to initiate rolling to supine.

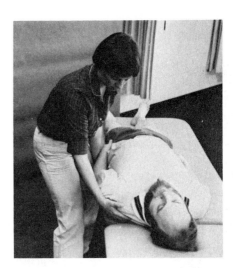

Therapist's hand position to complete rolling to supine.

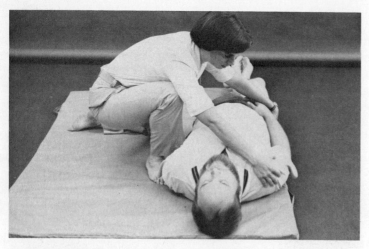

Starting position for turning on the floor mat.

TURNING ON THE FLOOR MAT

When turning a patient on the floor mat, the same steps are followed as when turning a patient on a plinth or bed. The therapist should position herself on the side to which the patient is going to be turned. A half-kneeling position should be assumed, with the "down" knee at the level of the patient's hips, and the "up" knee at the level of the patient's shoulders.

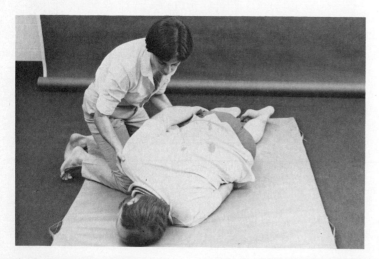

Turning supine to prone on the floor mat.

The therapist should place her left hand on the patient's right hip, holding the patient's right hand on top of the hip. The therapist's right hand is placed on the patient's right shoulder. The hand position must rotate at the midpoint of the roll, as described earlier.

The therapist must move with the patient in order to allow the patient to complete a full roll. The therapist moves out of the patient's way as he is turned, allowing the patient to complete the roll without rolling into the therapist.

Completing the turn from supine to prone on the floor mat.

TURNING SUPINE TO SIDELYING

In the sidelying position, the patient will remain resting on his side for some time. Therefore, adjustments during the procedure of rolling must be made. Sidelying can be achieved from either the supine or prone position.

When the patient is to be positioned on his left side, his initial position is supine and to the right side of the mattress or mat. The left arm is abducted to 45°. The right lower extremity is crossed over the left lower extremity at the ankle. The right hand is placed against the right hip, palm against the hip.

The therapist assumes a position on the side to which the patient is turning. The therapist's left hand grasps the patient's right hip, holding the patient's right hand between her hand and the patient's hip. The therapist's right hand grasps the patient's right shoulder. The patient is rolled until the sidelying position has been reached.

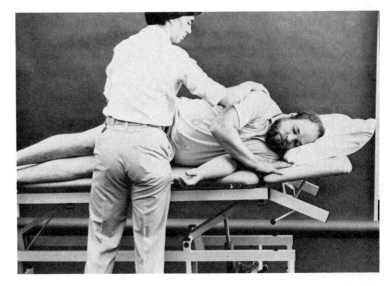

Turning to the sidelying position.

SIDELYING POSITION

The sidelying position requires a pillow under the head and if the patient is inclined forward, a pillow is placed in front of the patient. Then the uppermost arm is brought forward to rest on the pillow. If the patient is in a sidelying inclined backward position, the pillow is placed behind the patient, and the uppermost arm is extended and supported by the pillow behind the patient. The upper trunk may need to be rotated by bringing the lower-most shoulder forward. The uppermost leg is flexed and rests on pillows. To avoid excessive pressure on the bottom leg, the uppermost leg should not lie directly on top of the lowermost leg.

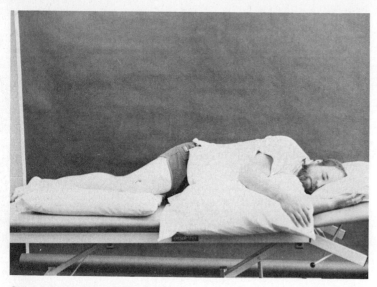

Sidelying position; inclined forward.

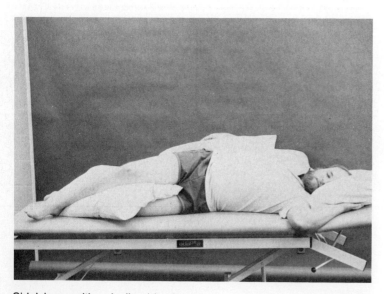

Sidelying position; inclined backward.

COMING TO SITTING FROM SUPINE

There are several methods for a patient to come to sitting from supine. The method used will depend upon the patient's functional abilities and the patient's medical problem. In all cases, a patient should not be left unguarded in the sitting position if he cannot maintain the position safely.

Illustrations include assumption of both long sitting and sitting upright on the side of a bed positions.

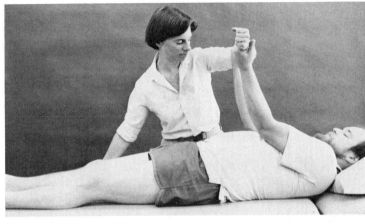

Sidelying position; inclined forward.

If a patient has enough strength, he can come to a sitting position by doing a sit-up in bed. If slight assistance is needed, ie, for a medical problem of general weakness, a trapeze bar can be used. In some cases a patient can use a sit-up or a trapeze bar while the therapist assists at the same time.

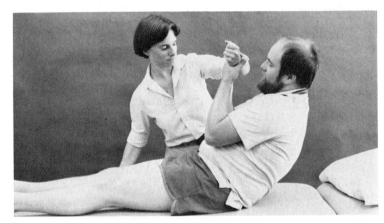

Midway up to sitting; therapist must move to allow patient to attain complete sitting.

To assist in the assumption of the sitting position, the therapist may put an arm behind the patient's back and push or pull to assist the patient. The therapist should be aware of putting too much pressure on an area of the patient's back, and should make sure the patient is able to maintain control during the movement and while in the sitting position. If a trapeze bar is not available, the therapist can stabilize her arm in front of the patient and allow the patient to pull himself up while pulling on the therapist's arm. The therapist should not do the patient's work by pulling her arm back as the patient holds onto the arm without pulling. However, the therapist must move in order to allow the patient to attain the full sitting position.

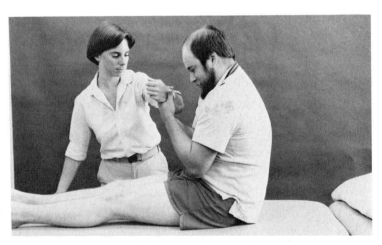

Completion of coming to sitting.

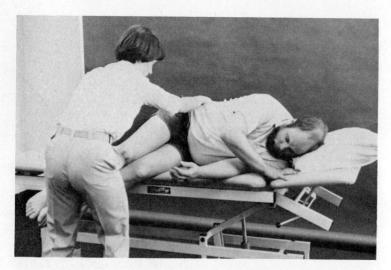

Lowering the legs off plinth in sidelying position.

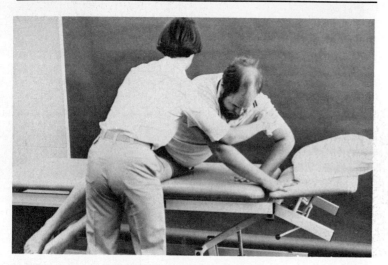

Pushing up to sitting with therapist's assistance.

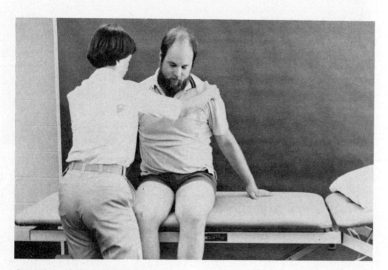

Attaining full upright sitting.

Another method of assisting a patient to the sitting position is to teach the patient to use his lower extremities as counterweights. If the legs are lowered over the edge of the bed, this will assist in coming to sitting. There are two ways of performing this maneuver.

The preferred method in which the patient can use the lower extremities as a counterweight is to start by assuming a sidelying position. This method is preferred because it reduces stress on the spinal and abdominal muscles and ligaments. The patient assumes the sidelying position and flexes the hips and knees to 90°. This places the lower legs over the edge of the bed. The patient can then push or pull himself to a sitting position. This maneuver may require a therapist's assistance.

An alternative method for the assumption of sitting on the edge of a bed from supine is used for some patients. This is necessary, especially for those who cannot move their legs or assume the sidelying position.

The patient pivots so that he is lying across the bed, the legs are then in a position to be lowered over the edge of the bed. The trunk should be raised at the same time as the legs are lowered. When necessary, the therapist can assist by putting an arm under the legs to assist leg lowering, by placing an arm behind the back and head to assist trunk raising, or both. Any of these assists will reduce the strain on abdominal and hip flexor muscles. For some patients who are too weak to pivot in bed, assistance may be necessary throughout the complete maneuver.

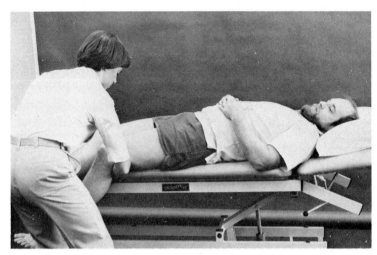

Pivoting on plinth to lower the legs.

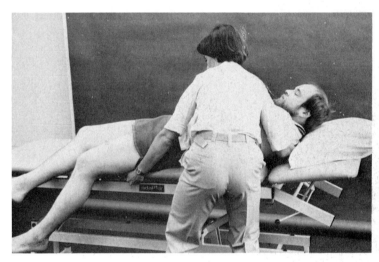

Therapist assisting patient to raise trunk.

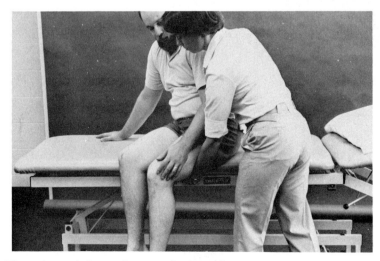

Therapist assisting patient to adjust position.

6
RANGE
OF MOTION
EXERCISE

INTRODUCTION

Range of motion exercises are movements of each joint and muscle through the range of motion available. Range of motion exercises are performed to prevent the development of contractures, muscle shortening, and tightness of adhesions in capsules, ligaments, and tendons that will eventually limit mobility. Each joint must be ranged in two different ways: (1) with respect only to its actual movement; and (2) with respect to the length of the muscles that cross the joint. Range of motion exercises also provide sensory stimulation which is beneficial to the patient.

Passive (PROM), active assisted (AAROM), and active range of motion (AROM) exercise may be performed. Passive exercise is usually used when the patient is unable to move a body segment. Some additional indications are when active participation produces increased spasticity or other undesirable muscle tone, produces pain, causes excessive cardiopulmonary stress, or concern for patient safety. In passive exercise, the patient is relaxed and the therapist moves the body segment. Active assisted range of motion exercise is performed when the patient needs some help to move because of weakness, pain, cardiopulmonary problem, or increased muscle tone. The therapist assists the patient to move through the available range of motion. Active range of motion exercises are performed independently by the patient, although they may be supervised by the therapist in order to insure correct performance.

When the therapist performs a range of motion, the body segment is held gently and firmly to provide support. The hand placement should allow movement of the body segment through full range with minimal hand repositioning. Support should be provided for all segments distal to the joint at which the motion is to occur. The movement should be of slow to moderate speed through all planes of motion available in a joint. Several joints may be put through range simultaneously, such as hip and knee flexion with ankle dorsiflexion.

Each joint should be moved through its full range of motion for both joint motion and muscle length. Joint range of motion is performed in order to maintain capsule and ligament length. To move a joint through its full range of motion, multi-joint muscles (muscles that stretch over more than one joint) must not be lengthened across all joints over which they act. Muscular range of motion is performed in order to maintain the length of muscles passing over a joint. To maintain the length of multi-joint muscles, they must be simultaneously lengthened across all the joints over which they act. Under certain circumstances, a goal of treatment is to allow multi-joint muscles to become shortened (not able to be lengthened over all joints at once) to a certain degree in order to provide a more functional length for that muscle. An example would be shortening of the finger flexors of a quadriplegic patient in order to provide some grasp and release as the wrist is extended and flexed. This is called tenodesis action.

Maximum range is achieved when the body segment cannot be moved further because of restriction by tissues or patient reports of pain. The "end feel" will vary depending on what is limiting further motion. When bone is limiting further motion, the end feel is hard (bony end feel). An example of bony end feel is when full elbow extension is attained. When muscle, ligament, capsule, or tendon tightness limits the movement, the end feel is soft (soft end feel). An example of soft end feel is when full elbow flexion is attained. When pain is limiting range of motion, the end feel may be empty (empty end feel). This occurs because there is no tissue limit to the motion.

In some cases, involuntary muscle contractions may interfere with range of motion. This can occur if a patient involuntarily contracts muscles to avoid pain, or in cases of upper motor neuron lesions. Muscle tone is altered in upper motor neuron lesions, and is felt in most cases as spasticity or rigidity. Spasticity is felt as gradually increasing resistance to movement, until a point is reached where further movement is prevented. This is followed by a sudden reduction of tone (clasp knife phenomenon) and movement through the remaining range of motion is then possible. Spasticity usually occurs in anti-gravity muscles. In the presence of spasticity, slow maintained movement will usually allow movement through the full range of motion. Quick movements will elicit the clasp knife phenomenon, or at least greater resistance to movement. Rigidity usually presents as resistance to passive movement in any direction. The resistance is the same throughout the range of motion. It occurs in both anti-gravity and pro-gravity muscles. Cogwheel rigidity, as observed in Parkinsonian patients, is alternating resistance and lack of resistance throughout the range of motion.

Range of motion exercises may be performed by moving the segment through each anatomical plane of motion separately, or by combining components of motion. The combining components of motion most commonly used are the diagonal patterns of motion of the proprioceptive neuromuscular facilitation[1] (PNF) approach to therapeutic exercise.

ANATOMICAL PLANES OF MOTION

All motions of the body are described in terms of starting from the anatomical position. The anatomical position is described as that position in which a person is standing upright, eyes looking straight ahead, arms at the sides with palms facing forward, and the feet approximately 4 inches apart at the heels with the toes pointing forward.

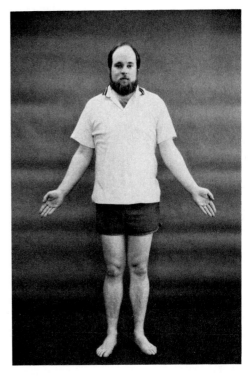

Anatomical position.

In the anatomical position, three anatomical (or cardinal) planes are defined. The sagital plane divides the body into two sides, left and right. The midsagital plane divides the body exactly into left and right halves. All motions called flexion or extension occur in the sagital plane. The frontal, or coronal, plane divides the body into front and back portions. All motions called abduction and adduction occur in the frontal plane. The only motions of flexion/extension and abduction/adduction that do not occur in their respective planes are in the thumb. Thumb flexion/extension occurs in the frontal plane, and thumb abduction/adduction occurs in the sagital plane. The transverse plane divides the body into upper and lower portions. All movements called rotation occur in the transverse plane.

The following definitions assume starting in the anatomical position.

Flexion: Except in the thumb, flexion is movement in the sagital plane. In the thumb, flexion is movement in the frontal plane. In the head, neck, trunk, upper extremities, and lower extremities other than knee and toes, flexion results in approximation of anterior surfaces. In the knee and toes, flexion results in approximation of posterior and plantar surfaces respectively. Dorsiflexion is the movement of the ankle that fits the definition of flexion.

Extension: Except in the thumb, extension is movement in the sagital plane. In the thumb, extension is movement in the frontal plane. In the head, neck, trunk, upper extremities, and lower extremities other than knee and toes, extension results in anterior surfaces moving away from each other. In the knee and toes, extension results in posterior and plantar surfaces moving away from each other respectively. Plantarflexion is the movement of the ankle that fits the definition of extension.

Abduction: Except for the thumb, abduction is movement in the frontal plane, and is the result of a limb segment moving away from the midline of the body. In the thumb, abduction occurs in the sagital plane, and is movement of the thumb away from the palm of the hand.

Adduction: Except for the thumb, adduction is movement in the frontal plane, and is the result of a limb segment moving towards the midline of the body. In the thumb, adduction occurs in the sagital plane, and is movement into the palm of the hand.

Opposition: Opposition is the approximation of the tips of the thumb and small finger of the same hand.

Internal rotation: Internal rotation is movement in the transverse plane in which the anterior surface of the limb segment is turned towards the midline of the body. Internal rotation may also be called medial rotation.

External rotation: External rotation is movement in the transverse plane in which the anterior surface of the limb segment is turned away from the midline of the body. External rotation may also be called lateral rotation.

Supination: Supination is movement in the transverse plane, and occurs in the forearm and foot. Supination of the forearm occurs when the upper arm is stabilized, and the forearm is rotated so that the palm faces anteriorly. Supination of the foot occurs when the foot is rotated about its long axis so the plantar surface faces the midline of the body.

Pronation: Pronation is movement in the transverse plane, and occurs in the forearm and foot. Pronation of the forearm occurs when the upper arm is stabilized, and the forearm is rotated so that the palm faces posteriorly. Pronation of the foot occurs when the foot is rotated about its long axis so the plantar surface faces away from the midline of the body.

Inversion: The term inversion is commonly used in place of supination. The technical definition of inversion[2] defines inversion as a tri-planar movement incorporating components of plantarflexion, supination, and forefoot adduction.

Eversion: The term eversion is commonly used in place of pronation. The technical definition of eversion defines eversion[2] as a tri-planar movement incorporating components of dorsiflexion, pronation, and forefoot abduction.

DIAGONAL PATTERNS OF MOTION

Two basic diagonal patterns have been described for each extremity.[1,3]. These patterns are modified by varying the position or movement of the elbow or knee, providing the ability to perform both joint range of motion and muscular range of motion. When combining components of motion are performed, the part may not be taken through as full of a range as when anatomical planes of motions are used. However, the mobility necessary for function is maintained. When the diagonal patterns of motion are used, the movements are performed simultaneously, thus the diagonal is achieved. The sensory feedback from movement in the diagonal pattern is thought to be closer to the sensory feedback provided by normal active movement. These are commonly referred to as D1 and D2, where "D" stands for diagonal, and "1" and "2" refer to specific diagonal patterns.

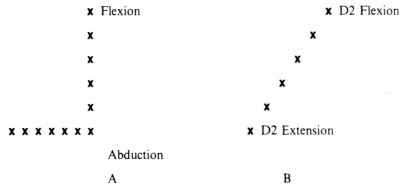

Combining components of motion, (a) separately; (b) simultaneously.

Table 6-1 lists the combining components of motion found in the proprioceptive neuromuscular facilitation patterns.

TABLE 6.1: Combining components of motion in pnf diagonals

DIAGONAL I UPPER EXTREMITY

	FLEXION	EXTENSION
Scapula	Elevation Abduction Upward rotation	Depression Adduction Downward rotation
Shoulder	Flexion Adduction External rotation	Extension Abduction Internal rotation
Elbow	Straight	Straight
Forearm	Supination	Pronation
Wrist	Flexed Radial deviation	Extended Ulnar deviation
Digits	Flexed Adducted	Extended Abducted

DIAGONAL I LOWER EXTREMITY

	FLEXION	EXTENSION
Hip	Flexion Adduction External rotation	Extension Abduction Internal rotation
Knee	Straight	Straight
Ankle	Dorsiflexed Inverted	Plantarflexed Everted
Toes	Extended	Flexed

DIAGONAL II UPPER EXTREMITY

	FLEXION	EXTENSION
Scapula	Elevation Adduction Upward rotation	Depression Abduction Downward rotation
Shoulder	Flexion Abduction External rotation	Extension Adduction Internal rotation
Elbow	Straight	Straight
Forearm	Supination	Pronation
Wrist	Extended Radial deviation	Flexed Ulnar deviation
Fingers	Extended Abducted	Flexed Adducted
Thumb	Extended	Opposition

DIAGONAL II LOWER EXTREMITY

	FLEXION	EXTENSION
Hip	Flexion Abduction Internal rotation	Extension Adduction External rotation
Knee	Straight	Straight
Ankle	Dorsiflexed Everted	Plantarflexed Inverted
Toes	Extended	Flexed

For each of the following passive range of motion procedures, we have indicated the joints being ranged, the motion required to perform that range, and the hand placement. For those procedures specifically involving multi-joint muscles, we have named the muscles being stretched. *The motions listed are the motions required to stretch the muscles, and are not the motions that the muscles produce.*

LOWER EXTREMITY

ANATOMICAL PLANES

Joints: Hip and knee

Motion: Extension and flexion

Hand Placement: Heel and posterior knee

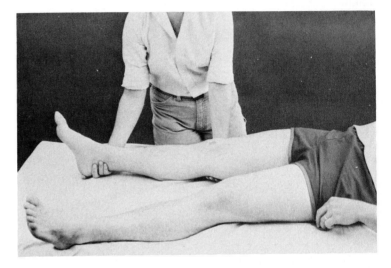

Hip and knee extension.

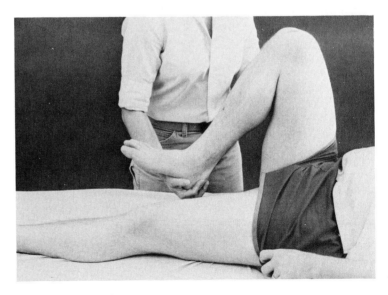

Hip and knee flexion.

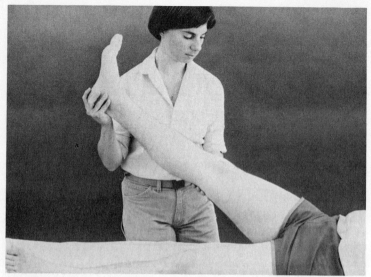

Hip flexion and knee extension, straight leg raise (SLR).

Joints: Hip and knee

Motion: Hip flexion with knee extension (Straight leg raise = SLR)

Muscles: Hamstrings

Hand Placement: Heel and posterior knee

Note: This maneuver is to lengthen the multijoint muscles of the posterior thigh across both joints over which they act.

Precautions: The knee must be kept extended, and the hip must be in the anatomical position.

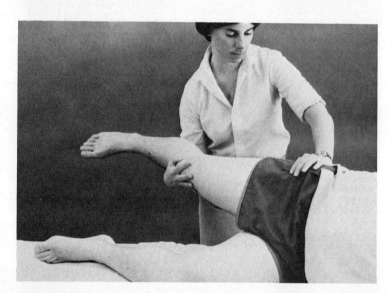

Hip extension.

Joint: Hip

Motion: Extension

Hand Placement: One hand is placed on the pelvis for stabilization. The other hand and forearm are used to support the patient's lower extremity in the anatomical position.

Note: The knee is maintained in extension.

Alternative Position: Prone

Joint: Hip

Motion: Abduction and adduction

Hand Placement: Heel and posterior knee

Precautions: Avoid hip flexion or rotation by keeping the knee and foot in the anatomical position.

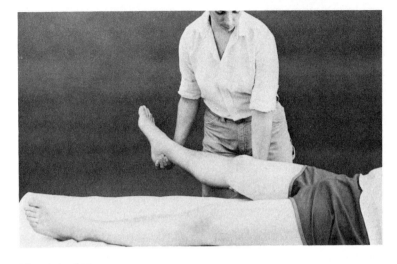

Hip abduction.

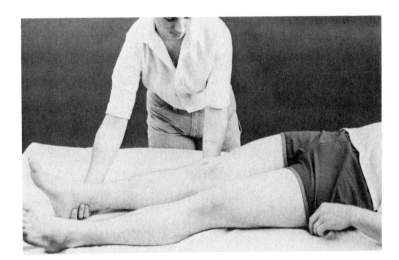

Hip adduction.

Joint: Hip

Muscle: Tensor fascia latae

Motion: Extension and adduction. The patient is sidelying.

Hand Placement: Ankle and lower leg

Note: The tensor fascia latae flexes and abducts the hip, and may assist in the extension of the knee. Therefore, hip extension, adduction, and knee flexion are required to stretch this muscle.

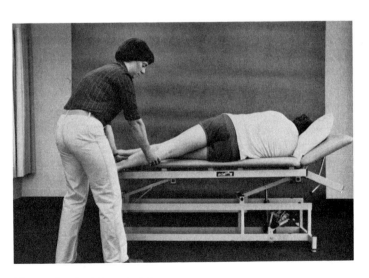

Tensor fascia latae stretch.

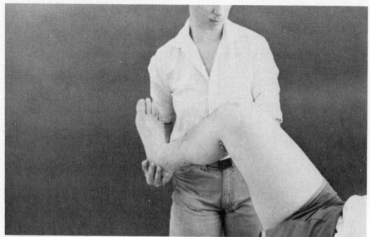

Hip internal rotation.

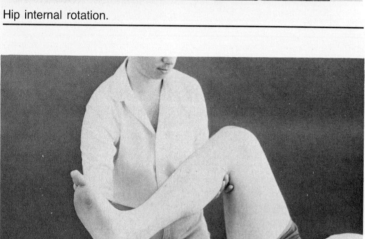

Hip external rotation.

Joint: Hip

Motion: Internal and external rotation. The hip and knee are flexed to 90°.

Hand Placement: Heel and posterior knee

Precautions: Avoid excessive stress on the medial and lateral structures of the knee. Maintain the pelvis flat on the supporting surface.

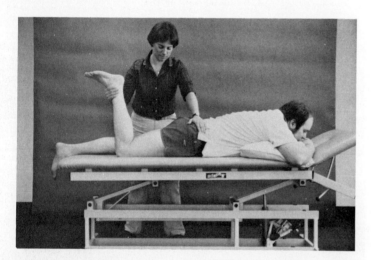

Rectus femoris stretch.

Joints: Hip and knee

Muscle: Rectus fermoris

Motion: Hip extension and knee flexion. The patient is prone.

Hand Placement: One hand stabilizes the pelvis and the other hand flexes the knee.

Precaution: The hip will flex if the pelvis is not stabilized.

Joint: Ankle

Motion: Plantarflexion and dorsiflexion

Hand Placement: Heel and dorsum of foot for plantarflexion. Heel and lower leg for dorsiflexion.

Note: To stretch the gastrocnemius muscle, the knee must be extended. To stretch the soleus muscle, the knee must be flexed so the gastrocnemius muscle does not limit motion. The force is applied to the heel in the inferior direction, and not to the ball of the foot.

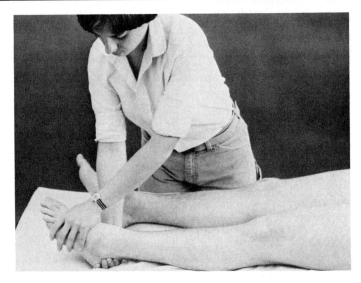

Plantarflexion.

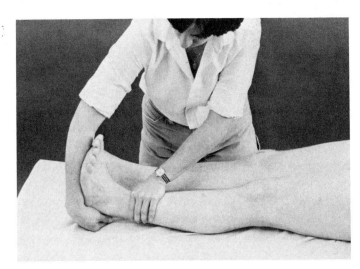

Dorsiflexion to stretch gastrocnemius muscle.

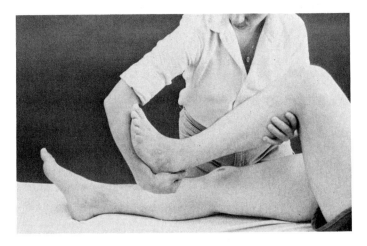

Dorsiflexion to stretch joint and soleus muscle.

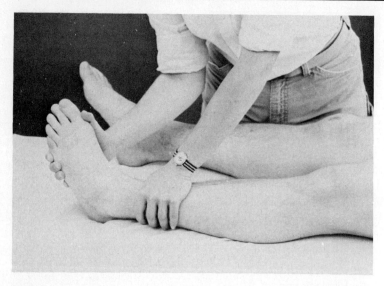

Inversion of the foot.

Eversion of the foot.

Joints: Foot

Motion: Inversion and eversion

Hand Placement: One hand stabilizes the lower leg and the other hand grasps the forefoot.

Joints: Toes

Motion: Extension and flexion

Hand Placement: One hand stabilizes the lower leg and the other hand grasps the toes.

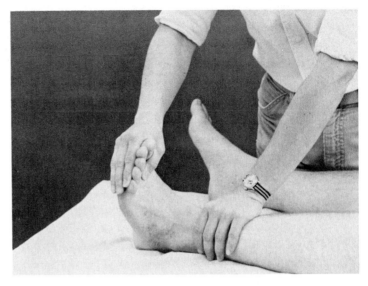

Toe extension.

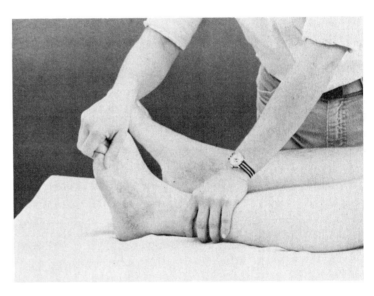

Toe flexion.

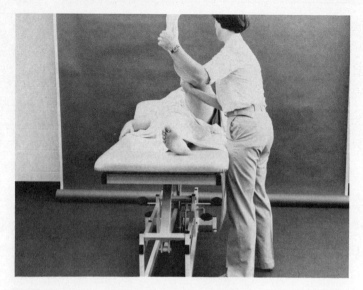

PNF diagonal 1 extension with knee straight

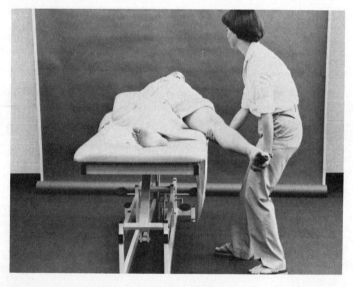

PNF diagonal 1 flexion with knee straight.

DIAGONAL PATTERNS

Pattern: PNF diagonal 1 (D1) extension with knee straight
PNF diagonal 1 (D1) flexion with knee straight

Hand Placement: Heel and posterior thigh

Combining Components: D1 extension-hip extension/abduction/internal rotation
knee straight
ankle plantarflexion/eversion

D1 flexion-hip flexion/adduction/external rotation
knee straight
ankle dorsiflexion/inversion

Note: Knee straight indicates that the knee remains in full extension throughout the movement of both patterns.

Pattern: PNF D1 extension with knee extension
PNF D1 flexion with knee flexion

Hand Placement: Heel and posterior thigh

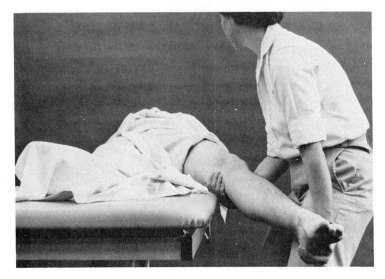

PNF diagonal 1 extension with knee extension.

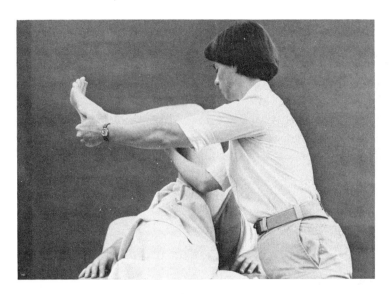

PNF diagonal 1 flexion with knee flexion.

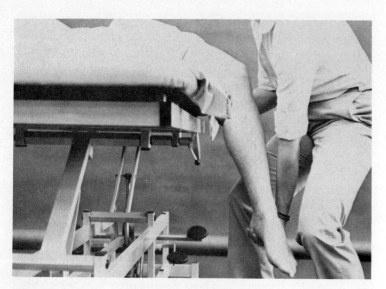

PNF diagonal 1 extension with knee flexion.

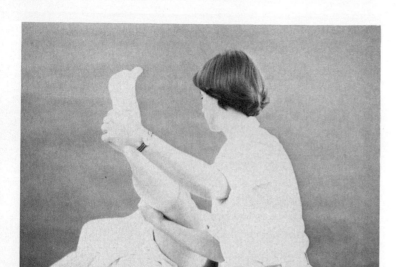

PNF diagonal 1 flexion with knee extension.

Pattern: D1 extension with knee flexion
D1 flexion with knee extension

Hand Placement: Heel and posterior thigh

Pattern: PNF diagonal 2 (D2) extension with knee straight
PNF diagonal 2 (D2) flexion with knee straight

Combining Components: D2 extension-hip extension/adduction/external rotation
knee straight
ankle plantarflexion/inversion
D2 flexion-hip flexion/abduction/internal rotation
knee straight
ankle dorsiflexion/eversion

Hand Placement: Heel and posterior thigh

Note: Knee straight indicates that the knee remains in full extenson throughout the movement of the pattern.

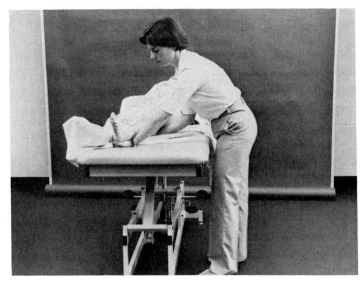

PNF diagonal 2 extension with knee straight.

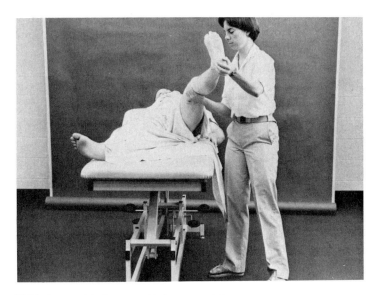

PNF diagonal 2 flexion with knee straight.

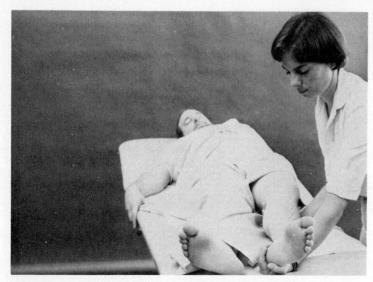

PNF diagonal 2 extension with knee extension.

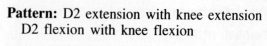

Pattern: D2 extension with knee extension
D2 flexion with knee flexion

Hand Placement: Heel and posterior thigh

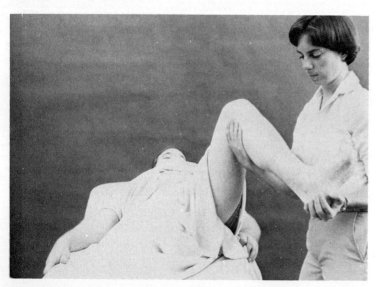

PNF diagonal 2 flexion with knee flexion.

Pattern: D2 extension with knee flexion
   D2 flexion with knee extension

Hand Placement: Heel and posterior thigh

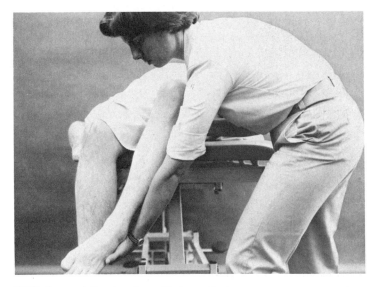

PNF diagonal 2 extension with knee flexion.

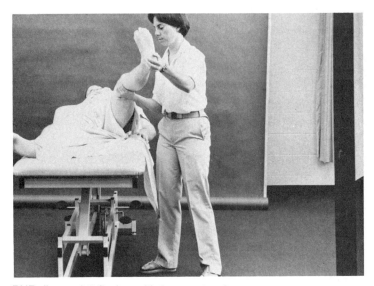

PNF diagonal 2 flexion with knee extension.

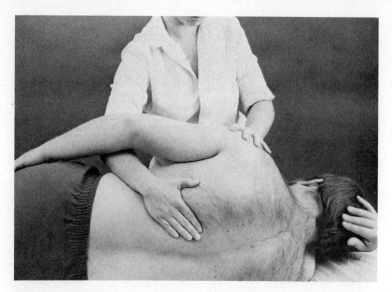

Scapular protraction.

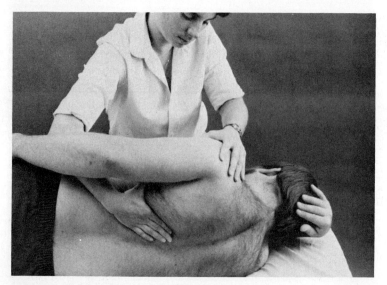

Scapular retraction.

UPPER EXTREMITY

ANATOMICAL PLANES

Joint: Scapulo-thoracic

Motion: Protraction and retraction

Hand Placement: One hand is placed over the acromion and the other hand is placed at the inferior angle of the scapula.

Joint: Shoulder (glenohumeral)

Motion: Extension and flexion

Hand Placement: One hand supports the wrist and hand while the other hand supports the upper arm.

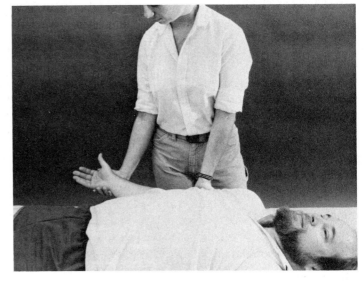

Shoulder extension.

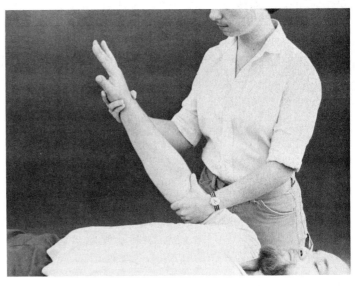

Shoulder flexion.

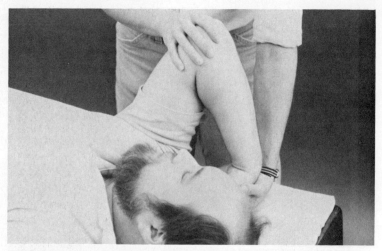

Shoulder and elbow flexion.

Joints: Shoulder and elbow

Muscle: Triceps brachii

Motion: Flexion

Hand Placement: The therapist supports the patient's wrist and hand with one hand, and uses the other hand to support the upper arm.

Note: To lengthen the triceps muscle across the joints over which it acts requires maximum flexion of both the shoulder and elbow joints.

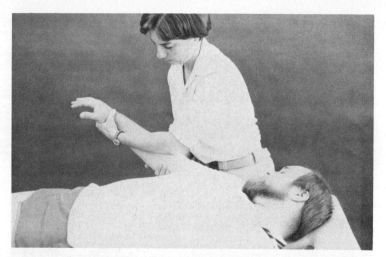

Shoulder and elbow extension; forearm pronation.

Joints: Shoulder, elbow, and forearm

Muscles: Biceps brachii and triceps brachii

Motion: Shoulder and elbow extension with pronation. Shoulder and elbow flexion with supination

Hand Placement: One hand supports the wrist and hand. The other hand supports the patient's upper arm. The therapist's left hand supports the patient's right wrist and hand.

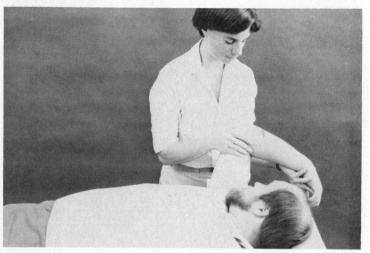

Shoulder and elbow flexion; forearm supination.

Joint: Shoulder

Motion: Abduction

Hand Placement: One hand stabilizes the shoulder girdle and the other hand and forearm support the patient's upper extremity.

Precautions: Avoid shoulder flexion and internal rotation during shoulder abduction. External-rotation must be permitted to avoid impingement. The therapist must move to allow full range of motion.

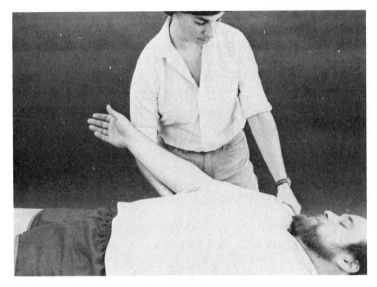

Starting position for shoulder abduction.

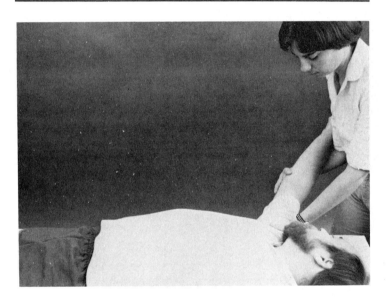

Completion of shoulder abduction.

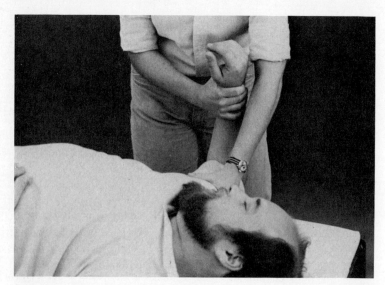

Starting position for shoulder adduction.

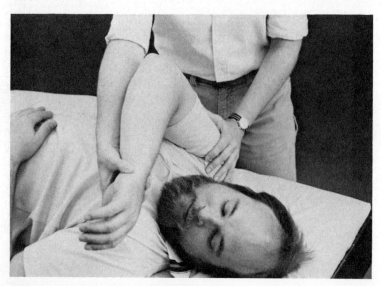

Completion of shoulder adduction.

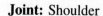

Joint: Shoulder

Motion: Adduction—the shoulder is abducted to 90° and the elbow is flexed to 90°.

Hand Placement: One hand stabilizes the shoulder girdle and the other hand grasps the forearm.

Joint: Shoulder

Motion: Internal rotation—the shoulder is abducted to 90° and the elbow is flexed to 90°.

Hand Placement: One hand stabilizes the shoulder girdle and the other hand grasps the patient's forearm.

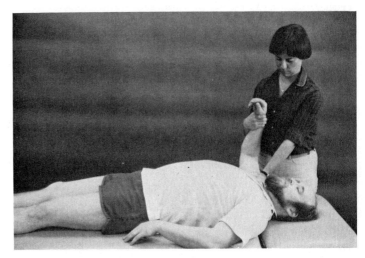

Starting position for shoulder internal rotation.

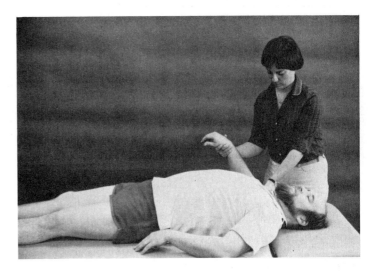

Completion of shoulder internal rotation.

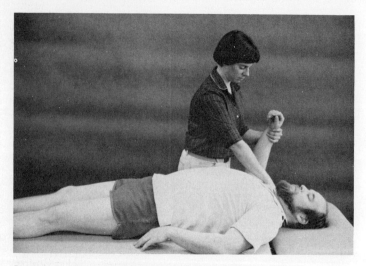

Starting position for shoulder external rotation.

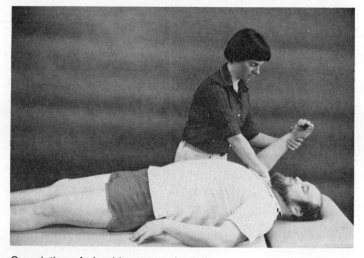

Completion of shoulder external rotation.

Joint: Shoulder

Motion: External rotation—the shoulder is abducted to 90° and the elbow is flexed to 90°.

Hand Placement: One hand stabilizes the shoulder girdle and the other hand grasps the patient's forearm.

Joint: Wrist

Motion: Extension and flexion—the elbow is flexed, and the fingers are allowed to move.

Hand Placement: One hand stabilizes the forearm and the other hand grasps the patient's hand.

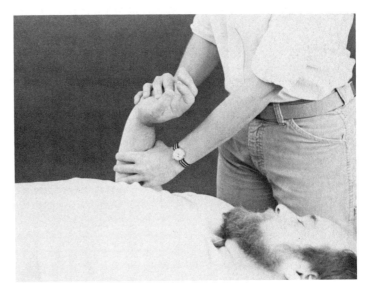

Wrist extension.

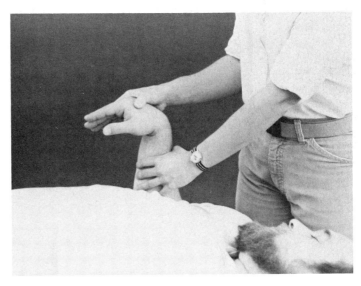

Wrist flexion.

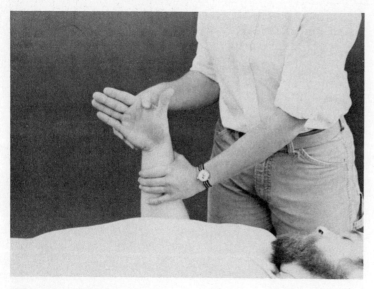

Wrist ulnar deviation.

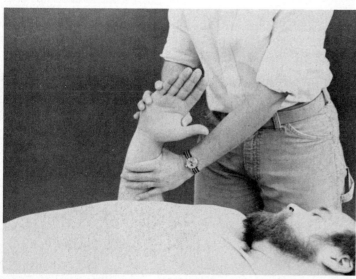

Wrist radial deviation.

Joint: Wrist

Motion: Ulnar and radial deviations

Hand Placement: One hand stabilizes the forearm while the other hand grasps the patient's hand.

Precaution: Avoid wrist flexion and extension while performing ulnar and radial deviation motions.

Joints: Fingers

Motion: Extension and flexion—the wrist is in the anatomical position and the elbow is flexed to 90°.

Hand Placement: One hand stabilizes the forearm and the other hand grasps the fingers.

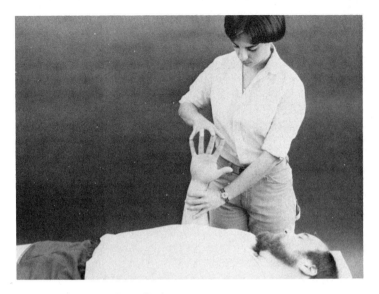

Finger extension; elbow flexion.

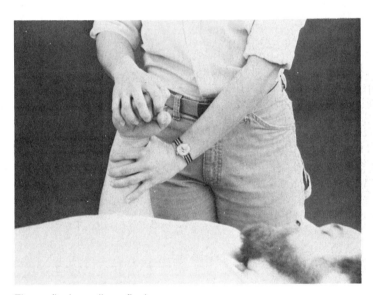

Finger flexion; elbow flexion.

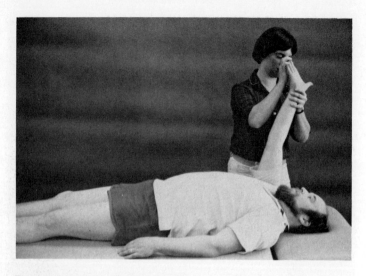

Finger extension; elbow extension.

Joints: Wrist and fingers

Muscles: Long finger extensors and flexors

Motion: Wrist extension with finger extension/Wrist flexion with finger flexion—the elbow is extended

Hand Placement: One hand grasps the wrist and the other hand grasps the fingers.

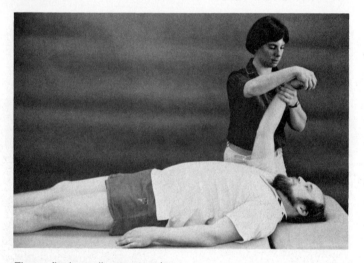

Finger flexion; elbow extension.

Joints: Wrist and fingers

Motion: Finger extension with wrist flexion/ finger flexion with wrist extension

Muscles: Long wrist and finger extensors and flexors

Hand Placement: One hand stabilizes the forearm while the other hand grasps the fingers.

Note: This position of the wrist allows the digits to be moved through full range of motion without stretching the multi-joint muscles of finger flexion and extension. This activity is performed to avoid loss of the grasping function that a natural tenodesis will provide.

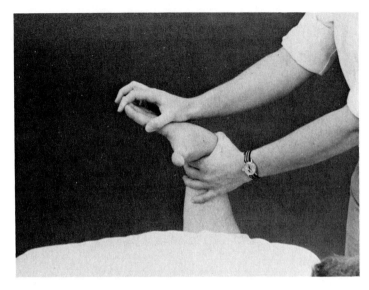

Finger extension with wrist flexion.

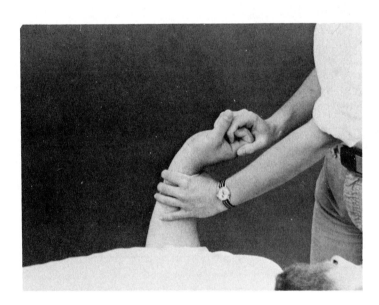

Finger flexion with wrist extension.

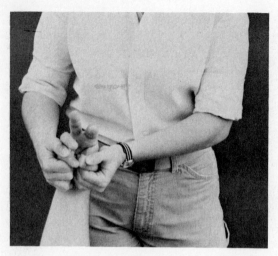

Thumb and finger opposition.

Joints: Hand

Motion: Opposition

Hand Placement: One hand grasps the thumb and the other hand grasps the fifth finger.

Note: In order to preserve the function of the hand, the arches of the hand must be maintained. Opposition of the thumb and fingers causes the hand to arch.

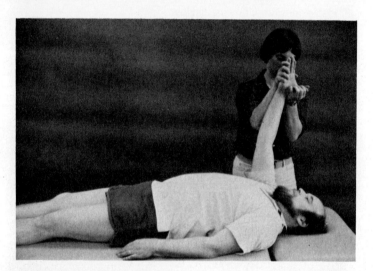

Stretch of web space of hand.

Joint: Thumb

Motion: Abduction—the thumb is extended

Hand Placement: One hand grasps the thumb and the other hand grasps the dorsum of the hand.

Note: Maintaining the ''web space'' is vital to a functional hand.

DIAGONAL PATTERNS

Pattern: PNF diagonal 1 (D1) extension with elbow straight
PNF diagonal 1 (D1) flexion with elbow straight

Hand Placement: One hand supports the upper arm and the other hand supports the wrist and hand.

Combining Components: D1 extension-shoulder extension/adbuction/internal rotation
elbow straight
forearm pronation
wrist extension/ulnar deviation
digit extension/abduction

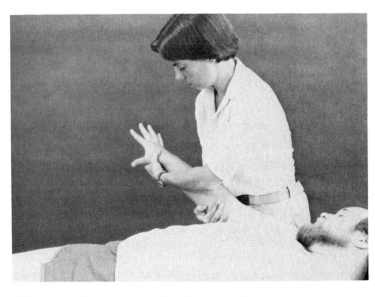

PNF diagonal 1 extension with elbow straight.

D1 flexion-shoulder flexion/adduction/external rotation
elbow straight
forearm supination
wrist flexion/radial deviation
digit flexion/adduction

Note: Elbow straight indicates that the elbow maintains full extension throughout the movement of the pattern.

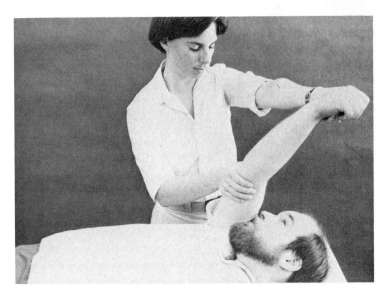

PNF diagonal 1 flexion with elbow straight.

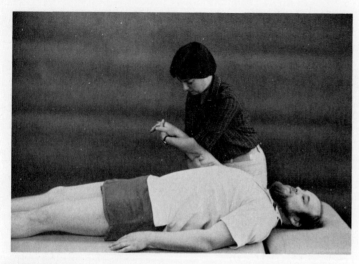

PNF diagonal 1 extension with elbow extension.

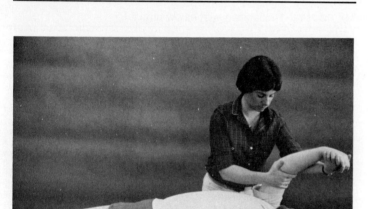

PNF diagonal 1 flexion with elbow flexion.

Pattern: D1 extension with elbow extension
D1 flexion with elbow flexion

Hand Placement: One hand supports the upper arm and the other hand supports the patient's wrist and hand.

Pattern: D1 extension with elbow flexion
  D1 flexion with elbow extension

Hand Placement: One hand supports the upper arm and the other hand supports the patient's wrist and hand.

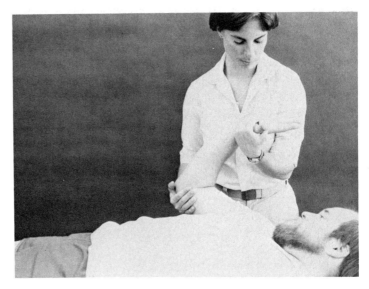

PNF diagonal 1 extension with elbow flexion.

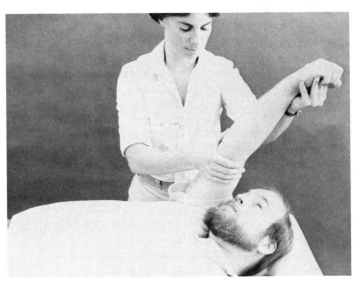

PNF diagonal 1 flexion with elbow extension.

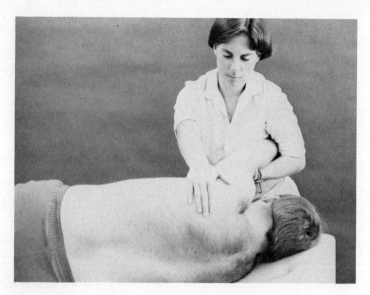

PNF diagonal 1 extension, scapular movement.

Pattern: D1 extension-scapular
D1 flexion-scapular

Hand Placement: One hand is placed over the scapula and the other hand and forearm support the patient's upper extremity.

Combining Components: D1 extension-depression/adduction/downward rotation
D1 flexion-elevation/abduction/upward rotation

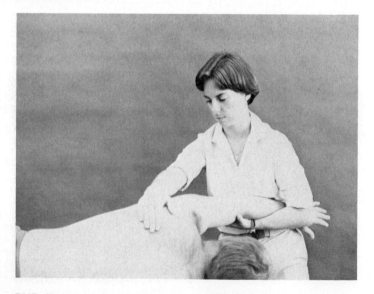

PNF diagonal 1 flexion, scapular movement.

Pattern: PNF diagonal 2 (D2) extension with elbow straight
PNF diagonal 2 (D2) flexion with elbow straight

Hand Placement: One hand supports the upper arm and the other hand supports the wrist and hand.

Combining Components: D2 extension-
shoulder extension/adduction/internal rotation
elbow straight
forearm pronation
wrist flexion/ulnar deviation
finger flexion/adduction
thumb opposition

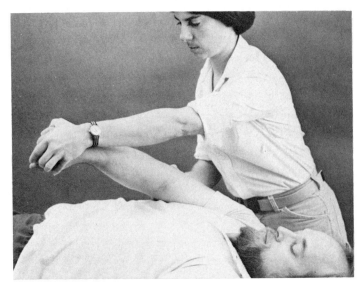

PNF diagonal 2 extension with elbow straight.

D2 flexion-shoulder flexion/abduction/external rotation
elbow straight
forearm supination
wrist flexion/radial deviation
digit extension/abduction

Note: Elbow straight indicates that the elbow maintains full elbow extension throughout the full movement of the pattern.

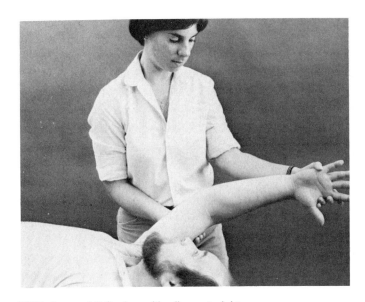

PNF diagonal 2 flexion with elbow straight.

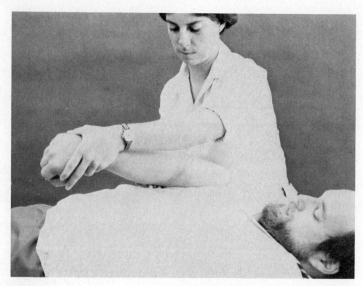

PNF diagonal 2 extension with elbow extension.

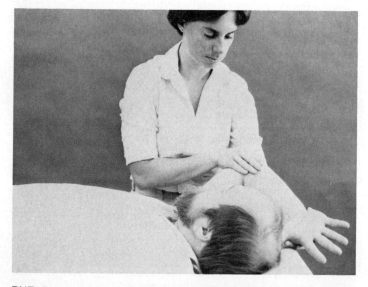

PNF diagonal 2 flexion with elbow flexion.

Pattern: D2 extension with elbow extension
D2 flexion with elbow flexion

Hand Placement: One hand supports the upper arm and the other hand supports the patient's wrist and hand.

Pattern: D2 extension with elbow flexion
  D2 flexion with elbow extension

Hand Placement: One hand supports the upper arm and the other hand supports the patient's wrist and hand.

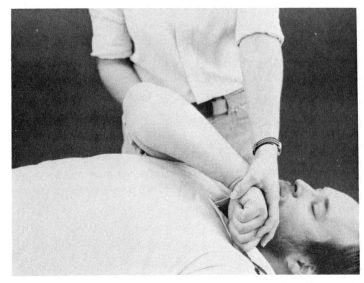

PNF diagonal 2 extension with elbow flexion.

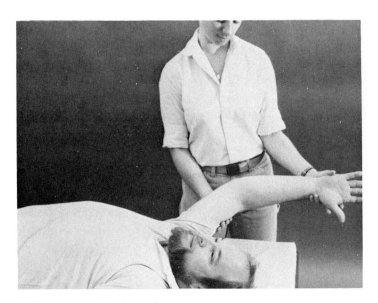

PNF diagonal 2 flexion with elbow extension.

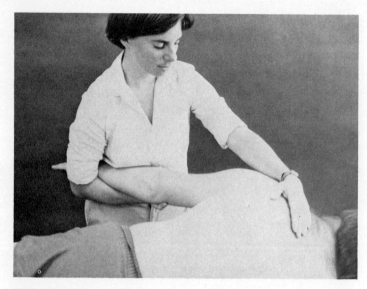

PNF diagonal 2 extension, scapular movement.

Pattern: D2 extension-scapular
    D2 flexion-scapular

Hand Placement: One hand is placed on the scapula near the inferior angle. The other hand is used to support the arm.

Combining Components: D2 extension-depression/abduction/downward rotation. D2 flexion-elevation/adduction/upward rotation

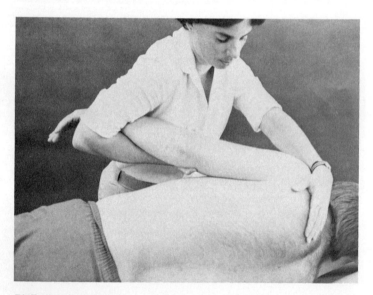

PNF diagonal 2 flexion, scapular movement.

REFERENCES

1. Knott M and Voss DE: *Proprioceptive Neuromuscular Facilitation*, 2nd ed.: New York: Harper & Row, 1968.
2. Warwick R and Williams PL: *Gray's Anatomy*, 35th ed.: Philadelphia: WB Saunders Co., 1973.
3. Sullivan PE, Markos PD, and Minor MAD. *An Integrated Approach to Therapeutic Exercise-Theory and Clinical Application*. Virginia: Reston Publ., Co., 1982.

7
WHEELCHAIRS

Wheelchairs are available in a variety of sizes and styles. Although wheelchairs generally have the same basic features, the mechanisms controlling the features vary. Familiarity with the common mechanisms and features allows for safer use and appropriate selection for a specific patient. This chapter illustrates basic features and some of the variations.

An important safety feature is the braking system. The toggle brake is engaged by pushing the brake lever forward. The brake is released by pulling the lever backward. The brake must be engaged whenever a patient is moving into or out of the wheelchair. A toggle brake may also be designed in the opposite directions.

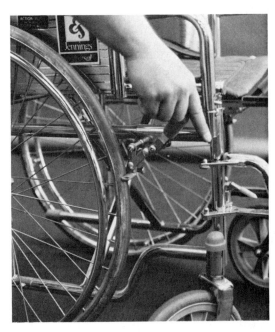

Engaging a toggle brake.

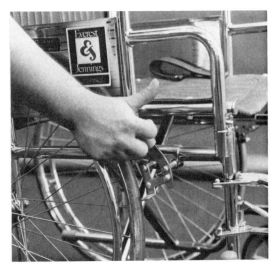

Releasing a toggle brake.

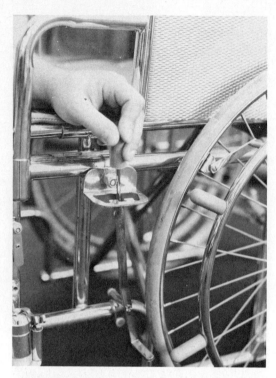

Ratchet brake.

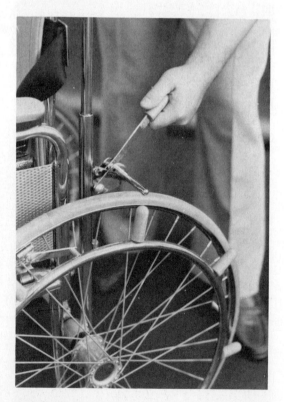

Additional brake on reclining back wheelchair.

The ratchet type of brake is also engaged by pushing forward and released by pulling backward. However, to maintain the brake in the locked or unlocked position, it must be slipped into the appropriate notch.

When a wheelchair has a reclining back, an additional brake is necessary. When the back is reclined, the wheel base is enlarged, altering the relationship of the brake and wheel so that the brake is ineffective. Attached to the back upright of the chair is an additional toggle brake operated by an attendant.

Another safety feature is a seat belt. Restraining belts are used to prevent patients from falling out of the wheelchair, and to provide trunk support. Some seat belts are attached or buckled in the back of the wheelchair so patients cannot release them.

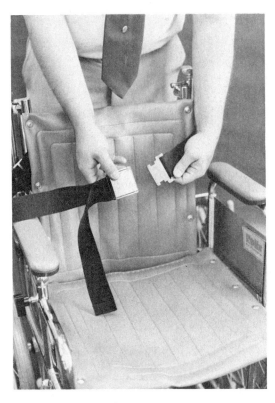

Seat belt for wheelchair.

The small front wheels are caster wheels. Two basic styles are available—the narrow, or standard, on the left in this figure; and the semi-pneumatic, on the right. The semi-pneumatic wheel provides some shock absorption and thus a smoother ride. The wider tire also makes travel easier on soft surfaces such as gravel and sand. A choice is made, and only one style is used on a given wheelchair.

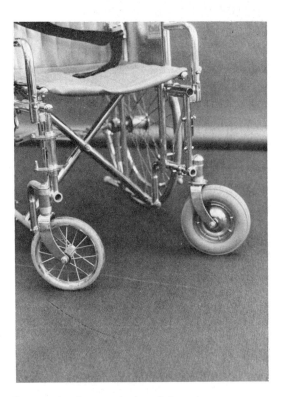

Caster wheels; standard on left and semipneumatic on right.

The large rear wheel may also be standard, ie, narrow and hard rubber, or pneumatic inflatable. The large wheel has an outer rim used by the patient to push the wheelchair. Many adaptations of the outer rim, such as projections, are available for use by patients who do not have grasp. Another aid in pushing on the outer rims is a non-slip coating to make grasp easier.

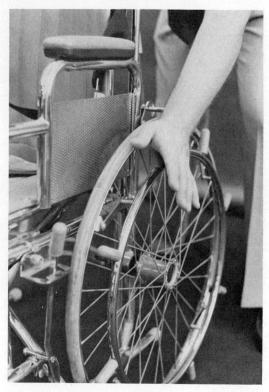

Vertical projections on push rim.

The pneumatic wheel shown here has two outer rims. This arrangement is useful in allowing a patient with only one functional arm and hand to push a wheelchair. The one-arm drive achieves forward or backward propulsion when both rims are used simultaneously. Pushing one rim at a time turns the wheelchair.

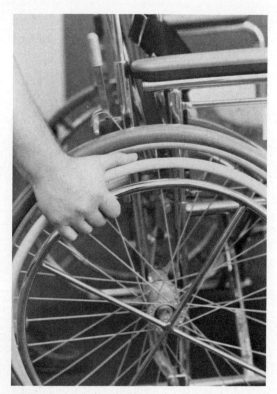

One-arm drive wheelchair.

Armrests are available in several styles. This figures shows a desk arm, so named because it allows the wheelchair to be rolled partially under a desk or table. Most desk arms can be removed and reversed so that the higher part of the arm is closer to the front edge of the wheelchair in order to aid in pushing to standing.

Several types of mechanisms are used to lock the armrest in place. The type shown here requires that a small button be pushed in as the armrest is lifted. Other types are released by pushing down on a small lever. Once released, the lever will remain down. Thus only one hand is required to remove the armrest.

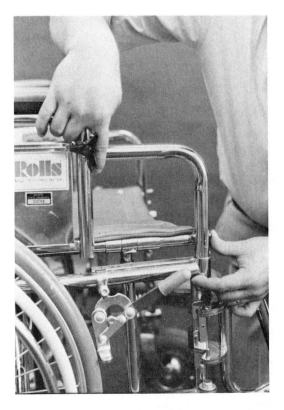

Desk armrest with pushbutton lock.

Another feature of some armrests is the ability to have the height of the armrest adjusted. The armrest shown here is adjusted by using the knob. In this way the patient can adjust the height of the armrests for different purposes.

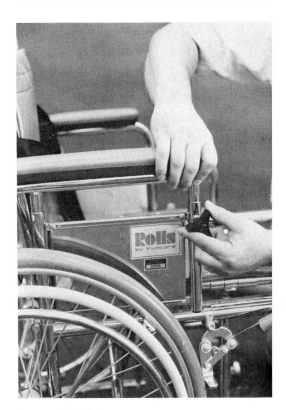

Adjustable height armrest.

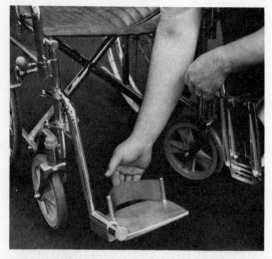

Footrest with heel loop in position for use.

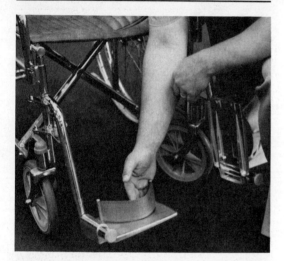

Footplate with toe loop forward.

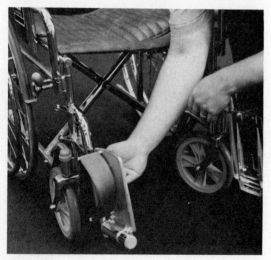

Footplate raised.

A footrest is standard equipment on a wheelchair. The footplate is available in several sizes to accommodate the patient's foot size. Heel loops prevent the foot from sliding off the footplate and under the wheelchair.

Toe loops may be used when the patient has difficulty maintaining the foot on the footplate in a forward direction.

The footplate may be raised to allow the patient to transfer safely in and out of the wheelchair. The heel loop must be pushed forward first to avoid being crushed and to allow the footplate to swing up completely. Avoiding crushing the heel loop also prolongs the useful life of the webbing. The footplate may then be raised.

Footrests may be fixed or removable. Removal may or may not require pivoting to the side. Several types of locks are used. This lock requires a downward force on the lever as the footrest is moved to the side. Lifting up on the released footrest allows the footrest to be removed.

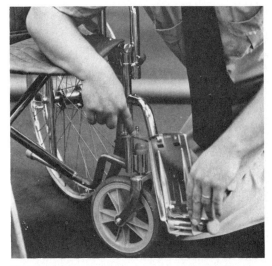

Pushing down on lever to release footrest.

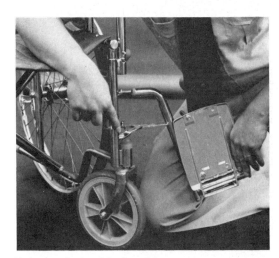

Swinging footrest to the side.

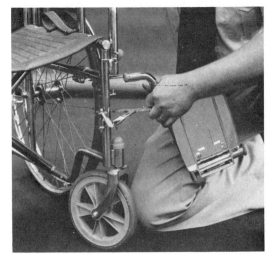

Lifting up footrest to remove.

Another type of release requires a forward force while pivoting the footrest to the side.

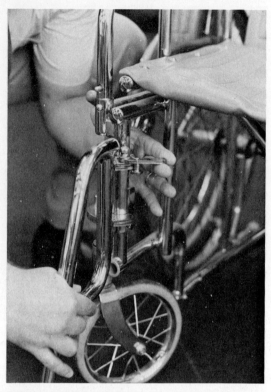

Pushing forward to release footrest.

The hinge for a swing-away detachable footrest is a simple design, as shown.

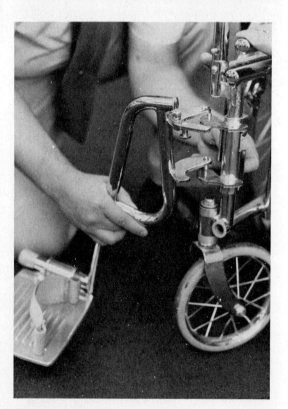

Hinge for swing away footrest.

An elevating legrest is most frequently necessary when the patient is unable to flex the knee or when a dependent position of the leg contributes to swelling. The elevating legrest can be adjusted in length to properly accommodate the full length of the patient's leg. A padded calf support is provided. The position of the legrest is adjusted by pushing down on the lever with one hand, while raising or lowering the legrest with the other hand. Elevating legrests can be detached from the wheelchair. Some can also be released and pivoted to the side so they are clear of the patient's feet during transfers.

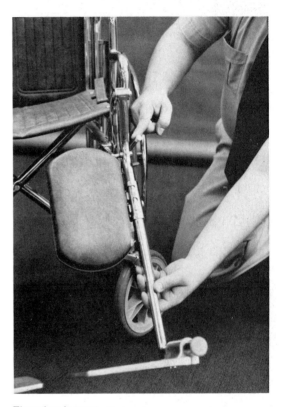

Elevating legrest.

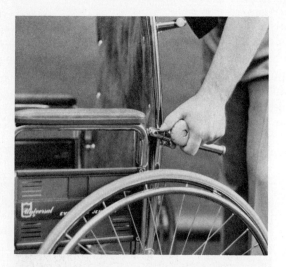

Releasing knob on back of semireclining wheelchair.

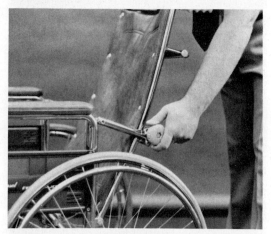

Tightening knob once backrest has been lowered.

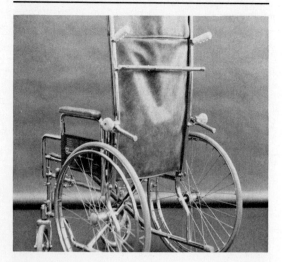

Semireclining back wheelchair with head support.

Reclining wheelchairs are available in several designs. The wheelchair shown here is semi-reclining. The angle of the back is adjusted by releasing the knobs on the side, raising or lowering the back to the desired angle, and tightening the knobs. A head support is required on a reclining back chair. The bar across the back of the wheelchair provides support and stability to the wheelchair.

Wheelchairs may be collapsed or folded for storage or transport. A standard wheelchair is folded by raising the footplates and pulling up on the handles located on either side of the seat. The wheelchair should not be folded by pulling up on the middle of the seat upholstery because this may tear the upholstery.

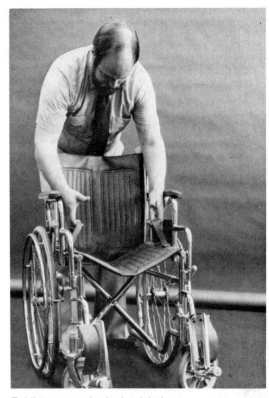

Folding a standard wheelchair.

To fold a reclining back wheelchair, the back support bar must be removed. The wheelchair can then be folded by following the same steps used when folding a standard wheelchair. The mechanism shown here is released by unscrewing the push handle.

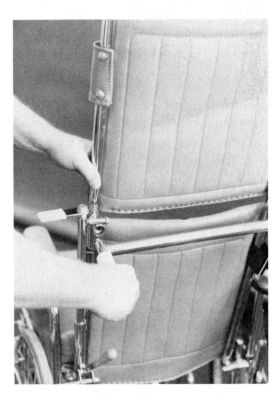

Releasing a reclining back support.

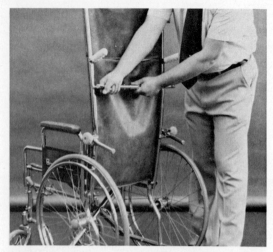

Starting to release a semireclining back support.

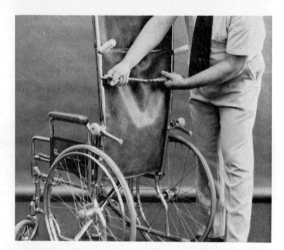

Completing release of a semireclining back support.

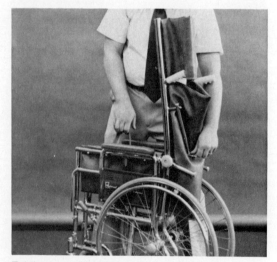

Folding a semireclining back wheelchair.

Another style of support bar is released by sliding the outer metal tube apart, revealing the hinge inside the tube. Pushing down on the hinge while the tube is pulled apart will release the hinge so that the wheelchair can be folded in the standard manner.

8
TRANSFERS

INTRODUCTION

Transferring a patient in or out of a wheelchair, bed, car, etc., may require the maximum assistance of several people, the minimal assistance of one person or no assistance at all. The patient should be evaluated, or a person knowledgeable about the patient's functional capabilities questioned, to determine the appropriate transfer prior to moving the patient. The safety of the patient and the therapist must not be compromised. Use of proper body mechanics will reduce the possibility of injury. The therapist must bend his legs and lift with the legs rather than the back. Positioning the feet in stride in the direction of the transfer will allow the therapist to shift and maintain control as the patient moves. The wheelchair, cart, bed, etc., must always be stabilized by securing the brakes, or by other means, ie, bracing against a wall.

Transfers requiring minimal, or no active, participation by the patient are called dependent transfers. Dependent transfers include the sliding transfer from cart to plinth, the three-man carry, the dependent standing pivot transfer, and the pneumatic lift transfer. Transfers requiring some patient participation are the two-man lift, the sliding board transfer, and the assisted standing pivot transfer.

The goal of assisted transfers is to reduce gradually the assistance required until the patient can perform the transfer independently. The assistance provided may be physical assistance with the maneuver, or verbal reminders of the steps involved.

Additional transfers include the wheelchair to floor and floor to wheelchair transfers. These transfers are necessary should the patient fall out of the wheelchair, or when the patient wants to participate in activities on the floor.

The patient should always be informed about the transfer and what he is expected to do. The explanation must be understandable to the patient. Commands and counts are used to synchronize the actions of all participants in the transfer. When the assistance of more than one person is required for a transfer, the therapist at the head of the patient gives the commands. The therapist explains how the command will be given; ie, ''I will count to three and then give the command to lift. When I say 'lift,' we will lift. One, two, three, lift.'' The therapist checks visually and verbally to insure that all assistants and the patient are ready before the transfer is initiated.

SLIDING TRANSFER—CART TO PLINTH

The cart should be positioned parallel to, and against, the plinth and secured.

The patient should be positioned to move towards the unaffected side.

When the patient can transfer predominantly under her own power, one person may assist by stabilizing the cart, and if necessary, providing assistance for the involved part.

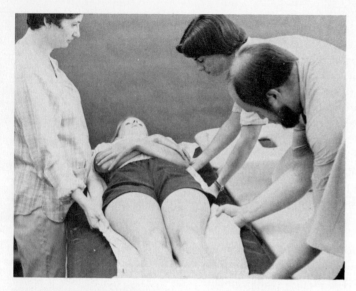

Ready to initiate transfer.

When the patient can provide only minimal assistance, three people are required to perform the transfer. The two people on the side of the plinth may not be able to reach over the plinth to lift the patient. They may kneel on the plinth and move off the plinth after the patient has been moved part way to the plinth.

The sheet under the patient is rolled and grasped close to the patient. A stronger grip is obtained by supinating the forearm.

The person at the head should be on the side to which the patient is moving. This person is responsible for coordinating the transfer by instructing the patient, determining when everyone is ready, and issuing the commands.

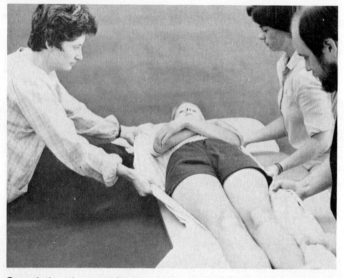

Completing the transfer.

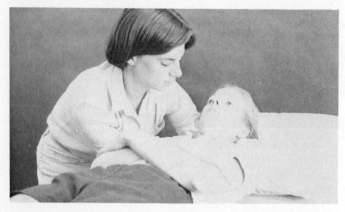

Cradling patient's head and upper trunk.

If the patient is unable to control her head and neck, the person at the head will support the patient's head by placing one arm under the head and the other arm under the patient's shoulders.

THREE-MAN CARRY

If the cart and plinth or bed cannot be arranged parallel to each other, or the sliding transfer is deemed unsafe, the three-man carry is used. The cart is positioned and secured at right angles to the bed, with the head of the cart at the foot of the bed, or the foot of the cart at the head of the bed. As the name of the transfer implies, three people are required to carry an average-size adult.

The three people involved in the transfer are positioned in such a manner that one supports the head and upper trunk, one supports the mid-section, and the third person supports the lower extremities. All involved place their arms beneath the patient so that the patient can be cradled from head to foot. The person at the head of the patient is responsible for instructing the patient, determining if everyone is ready, and issuing commands.

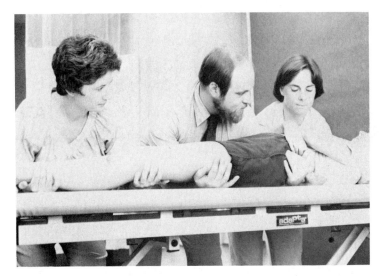

Starting position for three-man carry.

The transporters stand with their feet slightly apart and in stride. The knees are bent, and elbows are resting on the table.

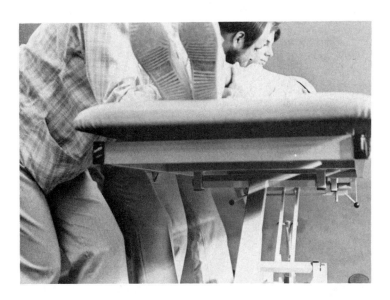

Starting position of transporters.

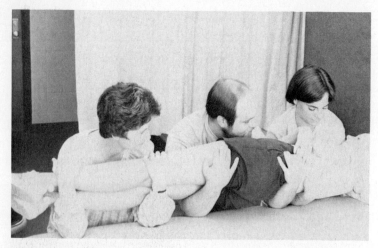

Cradling patient prior to lifting.

The patient is moved to the edge of the plinth upon command.

The patient is rolled onto her side in a log roll as the transporters flex their elbows. Thus the patient is cradled in the bend of transporters' elbows, bringing the weight of the patient closer to the center of the transporters' base of support.

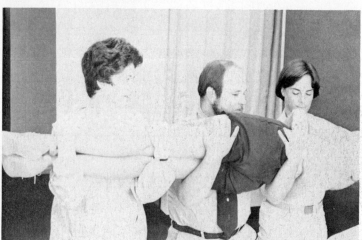

Lifting patient.

The transporters stand on command, lifting the patient.

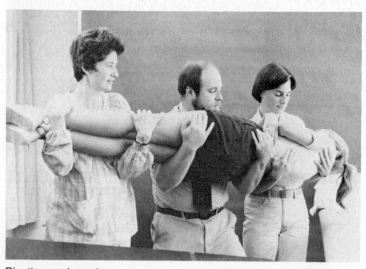

Pivoting and moving.

On command, the transporters pivot and move until they are all parallel to the cart.

Once parallel to the cart, the transporters again assume a stride stance, and lower the patient by bending their knees. The elbows of the transporters rest on the edge of the cart.

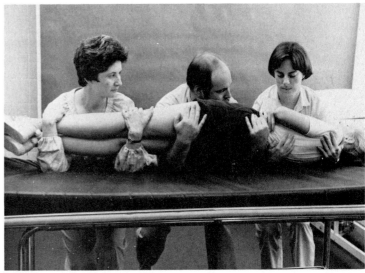

Lowering patient to cart.

The patient is uncradled as the transporters extend their arms. The patient is then moved to the center of the cart in proper alignment. The transporters then remove their arms carefully.

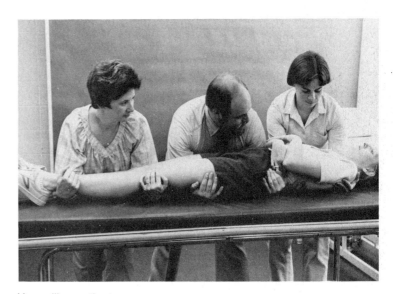

Uncradling patient.

PNEUMATIC LIFT TRANSFER

Pneumatic lifts provide a method for one person to transfer a dependent patient or a patient who is larger than the therapist. The pneumatic lift has caster wheels for easy positioning and moving. However, there are no brakes.

The base of the lift can be widened to fit around a wheelchair or other pieces of equipment. The base is in the narrow position when the patient is being moved in order to make maneuvering easier. The long lever attached to the base is turned and moved from one side to the other to increase or decrease the width of the base.

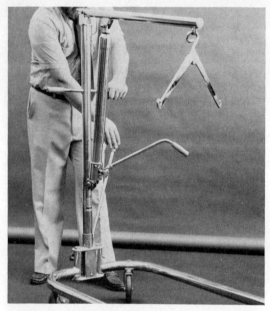

Narrowing hydraulic lift base.

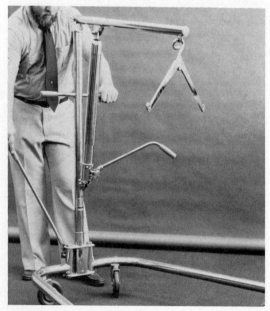

Widening hydraulic lift base.

The valve on the front of the upright is closed to allow the lift to be raised, and opened slowly to lower the patient. After checking that the valve is closed, the therapist pumps the handle to raise the lift.

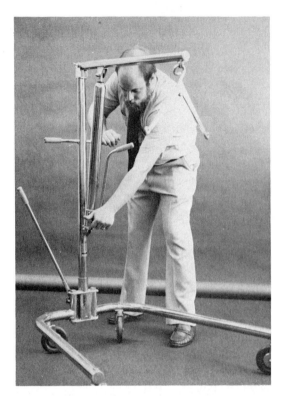

Checking hydraulic valve.

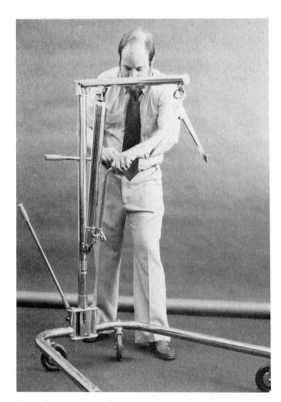

Pumping to raise lift arm.

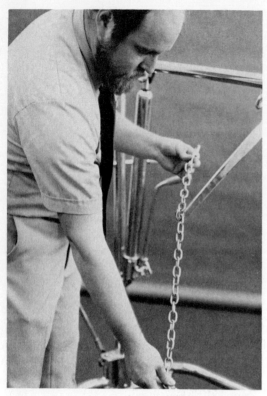

Chains attached to spreader bar.

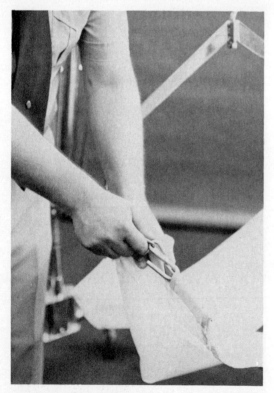

Attaching sling to chain hooks.

The sling on which the patient rests is attached to the spreader bar on the lift by chains. The length of the chain is adjusted to the height of the patient. A short segment of the chain is attached to the upper part of the sling, and a longer segment of chain is attached to the lower part of the sling to suspend the patient in a sitting position.

The hooks are attached to the sling from the inside to the outside. This will reduce the likelihood of the patient being injured by the hook.

The sling is positioned so the seams are away from the patient in order to avoid pressure areas.

Slings are made of a variety of fabrics. Some are one piece, and others are two pieces.

When the patient is in bed, the sling can be placed under the patient by rolling the patient to one side, positioning the sling, and then rolling the patient to the other side. The sling is left under the patient when in the wheelchair, thus the need to avoid pressure from the seams.

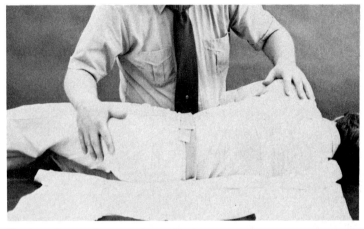

Placing sling under a supine patient.

Once the patient is positioned on the sling, the lift is moved into position so the spreader bar is across the patient. Both ends of each chain are attached to their respective sides of the sling. The valve should be closed, and the patient raised slowly. Care should be taken to ensure that a safe sitting position is attained as the patient is raised.

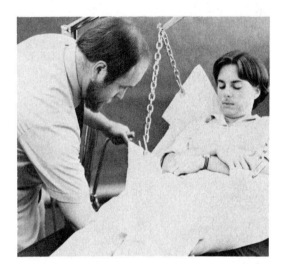

Raising patient.

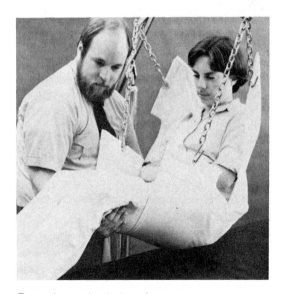

Removing patient's legs from cart.

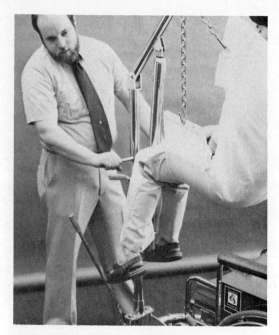

Maneuvering over the wheelchair.

The patient is moved into position over the seat of a locked wheelchair.

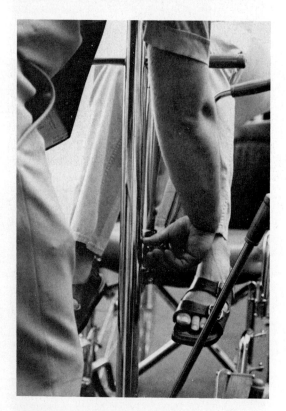

Opening hydraulic valve to lower patient.

The valve is opened slowly to lower the patient into the wheelchair.

Properly seating the patient in the wheelchair requires a slight pressure in the horizontal plane applied at the knees or thighs. This pushes the patient into the seat completely, with the patient's back resting firmly against the back of the wheelchair.

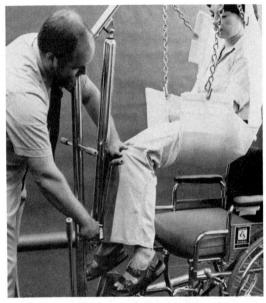

Pushing properly to seat patient.

Once the patient has been seated in the wheelchair, the valve is closed to avoid striking the patient should the lift arm continue to descend. The chains are then removed from the sling. The lift is moved away from the wheelchair, and the patient's feet are placed properly on the footrests.

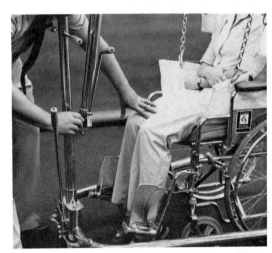

Closing hydraulic valve.

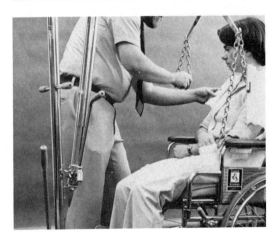

Removing chains from sling.

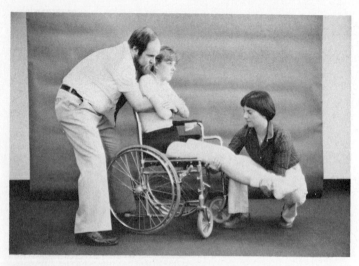

Starting position for two-man lift to floor.

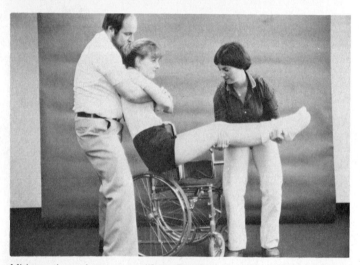

Midway through two-man lift to floor.

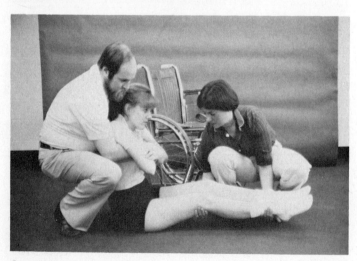

Completing two-man lift to floor.

TWO-MAN LIFT

When the patient has some upper extremity strength and trunk control, the two-man lift can be used. This transfer is often used to move the patient between the wheelchair and the floor.

To prepare the wheelchair for the two-man lift transfer, the patient's feet are removed from the footrests. The footrests are removed from the wheelchair if possible, or swung out of the way. The armrest on the side of the wheelchair to which the patient will be moved is removed.

The patient crosses her arms in front of her trunk. The therapist reaches under the arms and grasps the opposite wrists (left on right and right on left) of the patient. This prevents the patient from abducting her arms during the lift.

The therapist at the head of the patient places one foot on either side of the wheel, and leans around the handle. The position of the therapist may be modified depending upon the size of the therapist and patient, and the configuration of the wheelchair. The second therapist supports the patient's lower extremities by placing one hand under the thighs, well above the knees. The other hand supports the lower legs. The second therapist should have her feet in stride with hips and knees flexed. She faces in the direction of the intended transfer.

On command from the therapist at the head of the patient, the patient is lifted to a height that will insure that the patient clears all parts of the wheelchair. As a unit, the therapists step to the side or forward as appropriate, and then lower the patient. The patient is not released until she is in a position she can maintain.

To return the patient to the wheelchair, the maneuver is reversed. The armrests and footrests are removed as described previously.

The therapists start in a squatting, rather than half-kneeling, position. The half-kneeling position as the starting position would necessitate an extra movement into the squatting position. This would increase the risk of injury to all participants.

On command from the therapist at the head of the patient, the patient is lifted to a height that will insure clearing all parts of the wheelchair. The therapists step sideways or forward, as appropriate, so the patient is centered over the seat of the wheelchair. The therapist supporting the patient's legs should gently pull the patient's legs away from the back of the wheelchair in order that the patient will clear the upright of the back of the wheelchair seat. Once the wheelchair back has been cleared, the patient must be pushed towards the back of the wheelchair for the assumption of proper sitting posture.

When the patient is seated in a position she can maintain, the armrest and footrests are replaced, and the patient's feet are placed on the footrests.

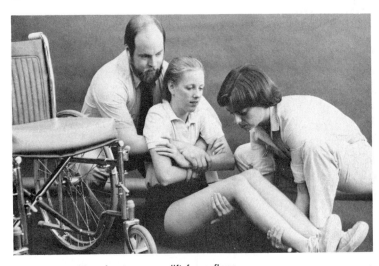

Starting position for two-man lift from floor.

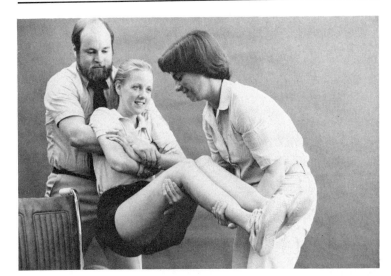

Midway through two-man lift from floor; clear the wheel.

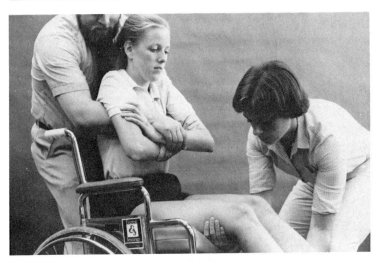

Completing two-man lift into wheelchair.

SLIDING BOARD TRANSFER

The sliding board transfer is used when the patient is not strong enough or lacks the sitting balance necessary to do a pushup transfer. The wheelchair is positioned and locked parallel, or at a slight angle, to the plinth. The patient's feet are removed from the footrests and placed on the floor. The footrests are moved out of the way. The patient scoots forward in the wheelchair, and the armrest on the side next to the plinth is removed.

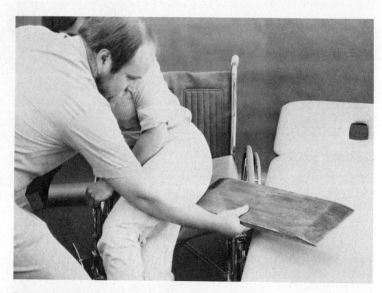

Positioning sliding board under patient.

The patient leans away from the plinth, and the sliding board is placed well under the buttocks. Care must be taken not to pinch the patient between the sliding board and wheelchair seat. The patient then moves back into an upright sitting position.

The patient performs the transfer by doing a series of pushups, lifting the body by straightening the arms and depressing the shoulders. The patient moves slightly towards the side of the plinth each time while lowering to the sliding board. The patient may place palms flat on the sliding board, or make a fist and place the outside of the fist on the sliding board in order to achieve a higher lift during the pushups. Some patients cannot lift high enough to clear the sliding board, and so slide their body across the sliding board. Hence the name, sliding board transfer.

As the patient gains the necessary strength, control, and endurance, the assistance of the therapist is decreased until the patient can perform the transfer independently. For many patients, the sliding board itself is then no longer necessary.

The therapist guards the patient by standing in front of the patient and blocking the patient's knees to prevent her from sliding forward and off of the sliding board. The therapist can provide assistance for lifting by placing his hands under the patient's buttocks, and lifting as the patient performs the pushup. When the patient needs assistance for balance, the therapist can assist by placing his hands on the patient's shoulders.

The patient can initially push on the remaining armrest to achieve a higher lift. The patient should be cautioned against grasping the edge of the sliding board, or the fingers may be pinched.

When the patient is on the plinth, the sliding board is removed. The therapist does not release the patient until the patient is in a position she can maintain.

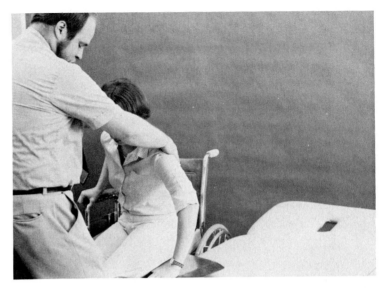

Beginning sliding board transfer.

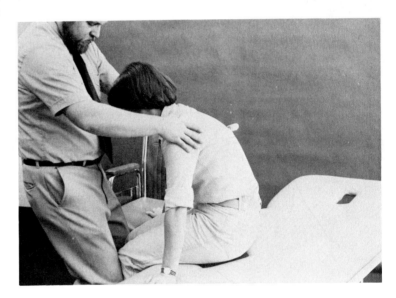

Completing sliding board transfer.

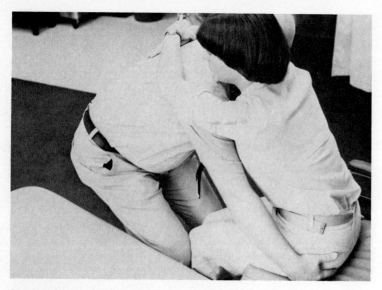

Starting position for a dependent standing pivot transfer.

DEPENDENT STANDING PIVOT

The wheelchair is placed parallel to the plinth and locked. The patient's feet are placed on the floor, and the footrests are removed. The armrest next to the plinth is removed. The patient is moved forward in the wheelchair to facilitate clearing the wheel. The therapist places his feet and knees outside of the patient's feet and knees. The therapist's hands are placed under the patient's buttocks. The patient places her arms around the therapist's upper back.

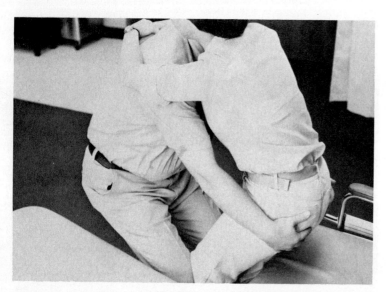

Lifting the patient for a dependent standing pivot transfer.

To synchronize the patient's efforts and the therapist's assistance, the therapist counts and gives commands. As the therapist counts, he initiates a rocking motion in time to the counts in order to develop momentum. On the command "lift," the therapist straightens his legs and lifts the patient from the wheelchair. The lift is only high enough to clear the wheelchair and any height difference between the wheelchair and the plinth.

The therapist pivots towards the plinth, rotating the patient to the proper position for sitting on the plinth.

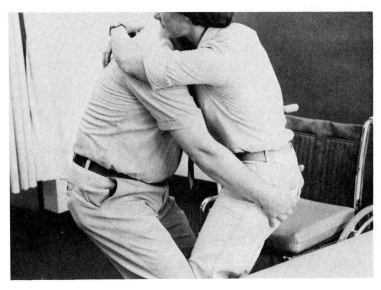

Pivoting the patient for a dependent standing pivot transfer.

The patient is lowered to a sitting position on the plinth by the therapist. The patient is not released until she is in a position she can maintain.

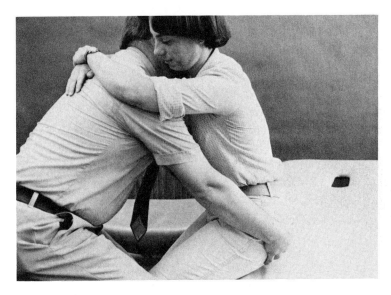

Completing dependent standing pivot transfer.

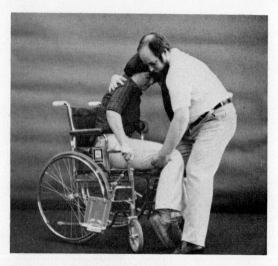

Assisting patient to move forward in wheelchair.

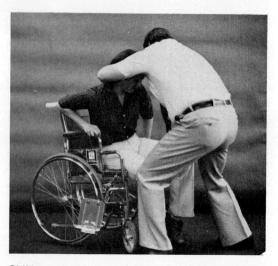

Shifting position to unload one buttock.

ASSIST TO FRONT EDGE OF CHAIR

The patient must maneuver to the front edge of the wheelchair seat. Sitting on the front edge of the wheelchair allows the patient to get her center of gravity over her base of support rapidly and easily as she comes to standing.

If the patient is unable to scoot forward in the wheelchair, the therapist can assist by placing one arm around the patient's shoulders to shift her weight off one buttock. With the other hand, the therapist assists the patient to move her leg forward by lifting under the thigh. The therapist then reverses his position and performs the same maneuver on the other side. This is repeated until the patient reaches the edge of the seat.

As the patient improves, assistance is reduced until the patient is performing the task independently.

An alternative method of getting the patient to the edge of the seat involves moving the pelvis as a unit and then the upper trunk as a unit. The therapist places both hands under the patient's buttocks and assists by lifting as the patient slides the buttocks to the edge of the seat. The therapist then places his hands behind the patient's shoulders and assists the patient in moving her shoulders forward.

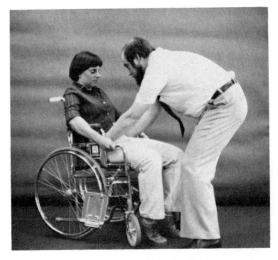

Assisting patient to move hips forward.

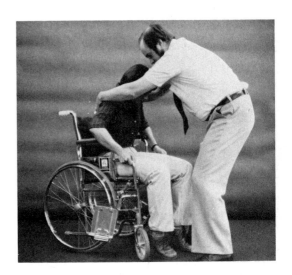

Assisting patient to move upper trunk forward.

ASSISTED STANDING PIVOT

The assisted standing pivot transfer is used when the patient can stand, pivot, and sit, but needs some assistance to perform these maneuvers safely. This transfer is also used to teach the patient to transfer independently. The therapist reduces the amount of assistance as the patient is capable, until maximum independence is gained.

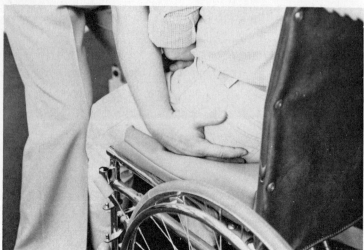

Hand placement under buttock.

The wheelchair is positioned and locked at a slight angle to the plinth. The patient's feet are placed on the floor and the footrests are removed.

To assist the patient in attaining the standing position, the therapist can vary the amount and type of assistance provided by varying the hand position. By placing a hand under the buttocks, the therapist can help lift the patient.

By placing a hand on the side of the pelvis, the therapist can guide the patient. The hand is in a position to control excessive lateral shift. From this position the hand can be moved posteriorly to support the patient if necessary.

Hand placement on side of pelvis.

With the therapist's hand on the anterior pelvis, he can guide or resist the patient's movement. Resistance may provide facilitation to make the activity easier for the patient, and teach the patient to bring her pelvis forward as she rises.

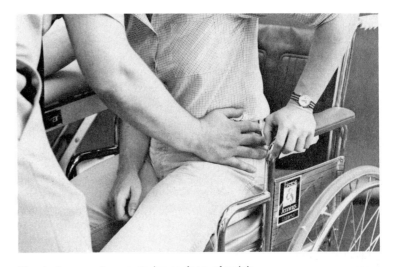

Hand placement on anterior surface of pelvis.

In the following examples of the assisted standing pivot transfer, the patient is role playing greater strength on one side, such as might be observed in a patient with hemiplegia. The patient must be able to transfer to both sides for complete independence. When initially teaching the patient to transfer, moving towards the stronger side is easier for many patients. Teaching the patient to transfer towards the involved side reinforces the patient's awareness and use of the involved side.

The patient is placed so she can move towards her stronger side during the transfer. The wheelchair is placed parallel, or at a slight angle, to the plinth and locked. The patient's feet are placed on the floor and the footrests are moved out of the way. The patient scoots forward to the front edge of the wheelchair seat, or is assisted if necessary.

If the therapist is unfamiliar with the patient's ability, he guards the patient's strong leg in order to insure support on at least one side during the transfer. The therapist always guards the hip and knee on the same side of the patient by having his knee in contact with the patient's knee, and his hand in contact with the patient's hip. This allows him to prevent the patient from collapsing at these joints. The therapist's other hand is on the patient's opposite shoulder to prevent the patient from falling to that side. In order to have a base of support in the direction of the transfer, the therapist is guarding the patient's left leg with his left leg. His foot is medial to her foot, so she will be able to move once she has attained the standing position. The therapist's left knee is lateral to the patient's left knee.

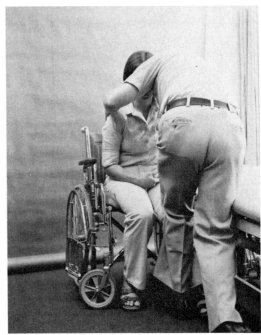

Guarding stronger leg; coming to standing.

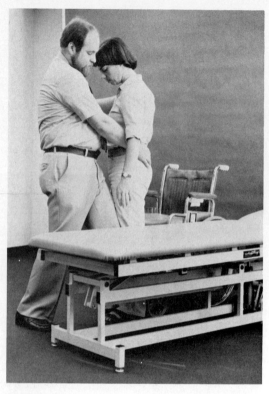

Pivoting.

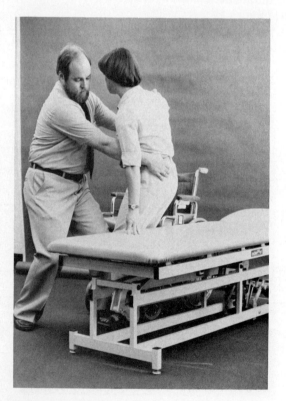

Patient reaching for plinth.

The patient pushes to standing using the arm of the wheelchair. The full upright position is achieved and is under control before the patient pivots or reaches for the plinth.

The patient pivots, and then reaches for the plinth. Reaching for the plinth before pivoting may lead to a loss of balance.

The patient is seated, and the therapist does not release the patient until the patient is in a position she can maintain.

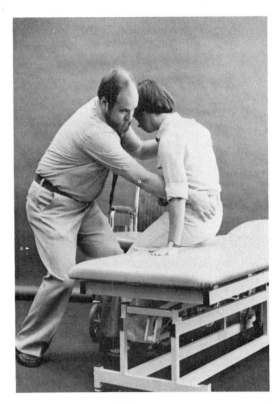

Patient sitting on plinth.

Once the patient has demonstrated ability to maintain the upright position using the strong leg, the therapist can concentrate on guarding the weak leg. Guarding the weak leg allows the therapist to evaluate the ability of the patient to use the weak leg during transfers, and to assist the patient to use the leg in a functional manner. The sequence of the transfer remains the same except that the therapist now guards the patient's right leg with his left leg. The therapist's left knee is in contact with the patient's right knee. The therapist's foot is lateral to the patient's foot, and his knee is medial to the patient's knee. The therapist's left hand is on the patient's right hip. His right hand is on the patient's left shoulder.

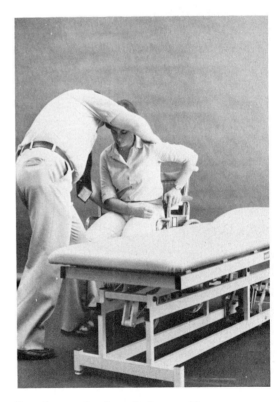

Guarding weaker leg; starting position.

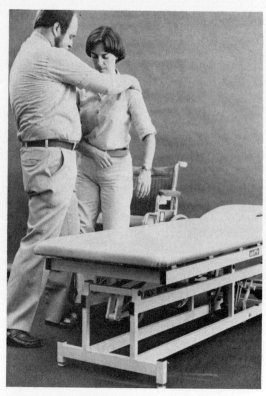

Attaining full upright posture before pivoting.

The therapist is in stride to allow him to move out of the patient's way as she comes to standing, and to move with her as she completes the transfer. The patient comes to standing by pushing on the arm of the wheelchair.

The patient attains the full upright position, and achieves control in this posture before pivoting.

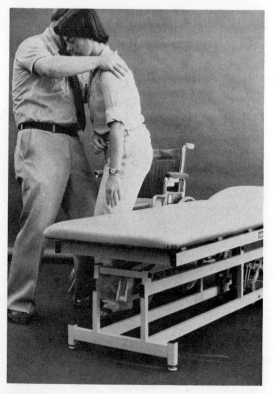

Pivoting.

The patient reaches for the plinth and sits.

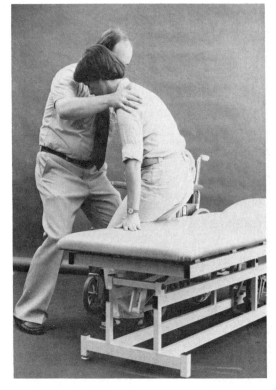

Sitting on plinth

The therapist does not release the patient until the patient can maintain this position.

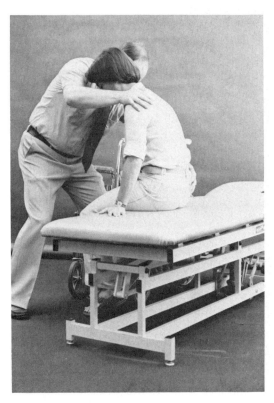

Reaching for plinth.

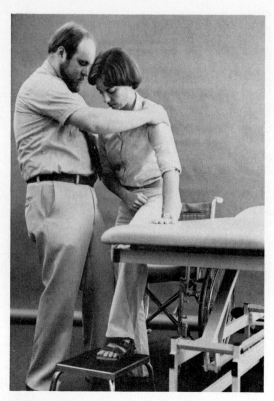

Stepping up on stool.

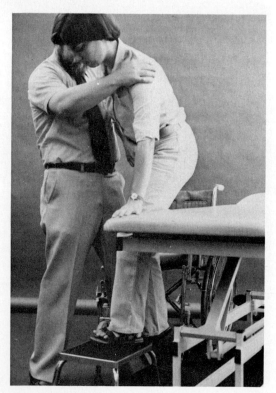

Lifting body over stool and pivoting.

Transferring a patient to a high plinth will require the use of a step stool, especially if the patient is short. The position of the wheelchair, guarding techniques, and the activity of coming to standing are performed as in the assisted standing pivot transfer.

The step stool must be in place before the patient stands. It is placed in front of the patient, alongside the plinth. With her hand on the plinth, the patient steps onto the stool with her stronger leg. The therapist must carefully guard the weaker leg in order to insure adequate support as the patient lifts and places her strong foot on the stool.

The patient straightens her leg in order to lift her body over the stool. This raises the pelvis above the level of the plinth.

The patient then pivots on the stool and sits on the plinth.

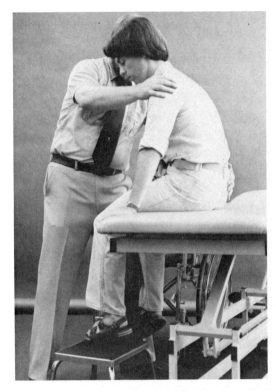

Sitting.

If the patient sits on the edge of the plinth and is unable to scoot backward, the therapist can assist by using a reversal of the maneuver he used to move the patient forward in the wheelchair. The only difference is that he assists the patient in pulling the thigh backward rather than pushing the thigh forward. The therapist must also guard against the possibility of the patient sliding off the plinth as the patient's weight is shifted onto one buttock.

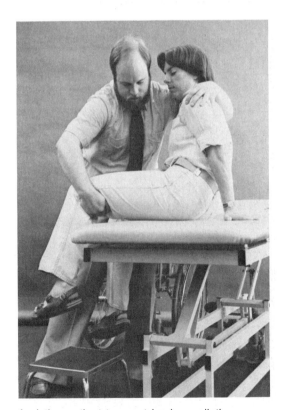

Assisting patient to scoot back on plinth.

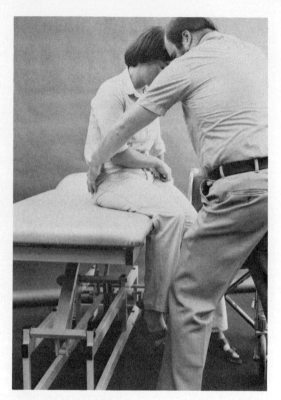

Lowering off of plinth.

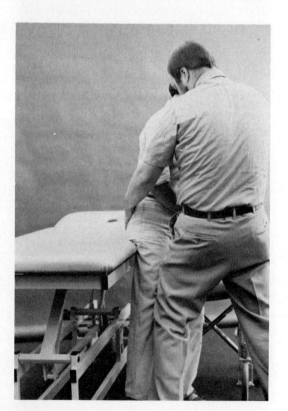

Attaining full upright posture before pivoting.

To prepare for returning to the wheel-chair from the plinth, the wheelchair is positioned and locked on the patient's strong side. This requires that the wheelchair be faced in the opposite direction, but on the same side of the plinth as used when transferring from the wheelchair to the plinth. To alight from a high plinth, a stool is not necessary. The therapist guards the weak side as the patient slowly slides off the plinth onto the strong leg.

From this point in the transfer, the remainder of the steps and instructions are the same, whether the patient is transferring from a high plinth to a wheelchair, from a low plinth to a wheelchair, or from a wheelchair to a plinth. The therapist usually guards the same lower extremity, and uses the same hand placement that was used in transferring from the wheelchair to the plinth. The patient attains full control of the upright posture before pivoting. After pivoting, the patient reaches for the armrest and sits. The therapist does not release the patient until the patient can maintain the sitting position.

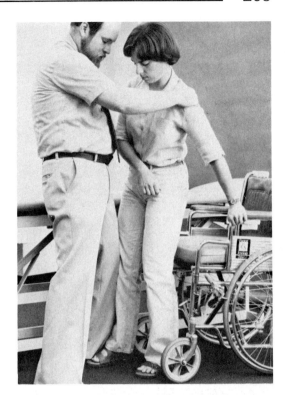

Pivoting and reaching for wheelchair.

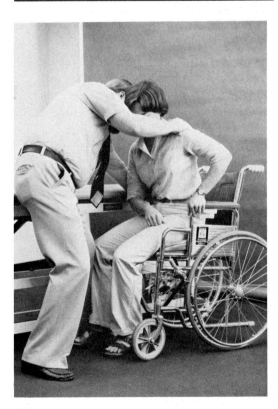

Sitting.

ONE-MAN TRANSFER FROM FLOOR TO WHEELCHAIR

Occasionally a patient may fall out of, or tip over, the wheelchair. If the patient is unable to transfer from the floor to the wheelchair, the family will need to be able to perform a two-man lift transfer and the one-man transfer. The two-man lift transfer is preferred because it is safer for the patient and the family members involved.

When using the one-man transfer, the wheelchair is positioned on its back, at the patient's feet. The patient's lower extremities are flexed at the hips and knees, and is moved so that the ankles are placed over the front edge of the wheelchair seat. The therapist performs a series of short lift and scooting maneuvers to move the patient into the wheelchair. To do this, the therapist places one arm under the knees and the other arm under the upper trunk and neck.

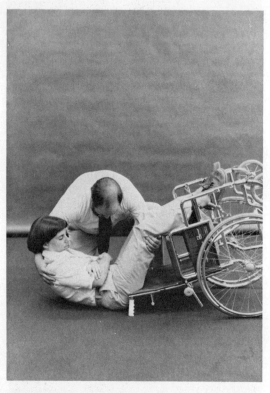

Lifting patient into wheelchair.

The therapist places himself in a half-kneeling position in order to provide a stronger lifting posture. The therapist then grasps the handles and lifts the wheelchair, bringing the wheelchair to the upright position as he moves out of the half-kneeling position to the standing position.

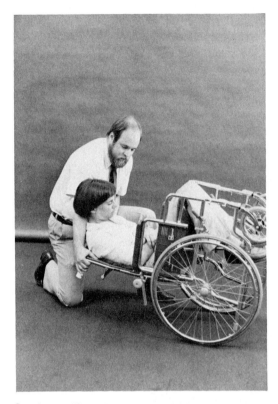

Starting to lift patient and wheelchair.

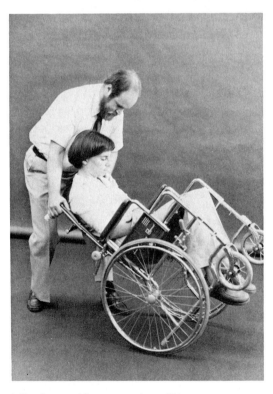

Adjusting position to continue lifting.

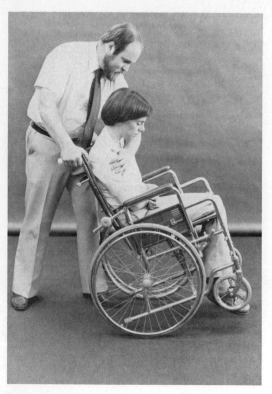

Supporting upper trunk.

As the wheelchair approaches the upright position, the therapist shifts one arm to guard the patient's upper trunk, in order to prevent her from falling forward.

INDEPENDENT TRANSFER FROM WHEELCHAIR TO FLOOR AND RETURN

INTRODUCTION

Many patients can, and must, learn to move safely from their wheelchair to the floor and back into the wheelchair.

The wheelchair is locked as the first step of any transfer. The patient's feet are placed on the floor, and the footrests are usually removed or pivoted to the side to avoid injury and allow more room for movement. The casters are turned forward, as illustrated below, to increase the base of support of the wheelchair. If the casters are not properly positioned, the wheelchair may tip forward as the patient scoots forward.

The method selected depends upon the strength, range of motion, and agility of the patient. The forward lowering to the floor and the backward lift into the wheelchair require the most strength and agility.

During training, the patient must be guarded and assisted to prevent injury or bruising that may result in skin breakdown.

The therapist is not pictured in the remaining photographs in this chapter to avoid obstructing the view of the patient.

FORWARD LOWERING TO FLOOR

The wheelchair is placed in the desired position and locked. The footrests are removed or swung to the side. The patient moves to the front edge of the wheelchair seat, and the legs are positioned in extension.

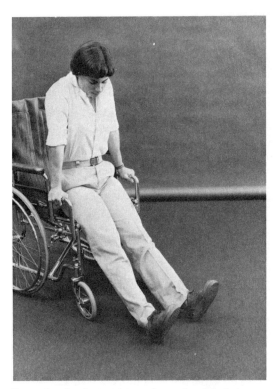

Preparing for forward lowering; wheelchair to floor.

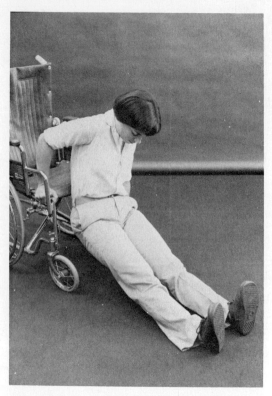

Re-positioning hands and starting lowering.

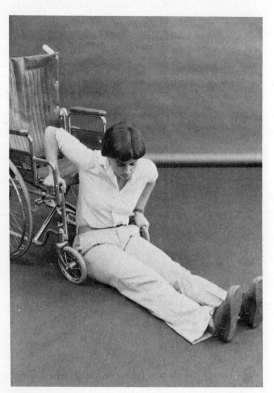

Sitting on floor.

One hand is positioned on the seat of the wheelchair. The other hand is placed on the caster or floor, depending upon the length of the patient's arm, strength, and range of motion. The patient then lowers herself to the floor.

BACKWARD LIFT TO WHEELCHAIR

The wheelchair is properly positioned with the caster wheels forward and is locked. The footrests are removed or swung out of the way. The patient assumes the long sitting position with her back against the front edge of the wheelchair. One hand is placed on the side edge of the wheelchair seat, and the other hand is placed on the caster or floor.

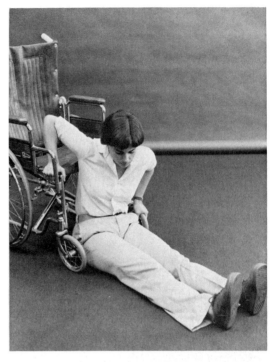

Starting position; backward lift to wheelchair from floor.

The patient pushes up by extending her arms and depressing her shoulder girdle, balancing on the arm holding the edge of the seat, then quickly moves the other hand from the caster to the armrest.

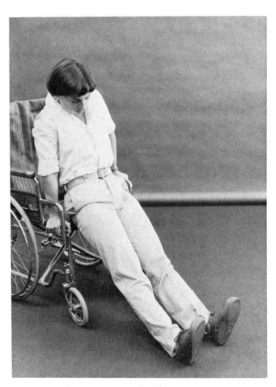

Initiating lift and repositioning hand.

Using the hand already on the armrest for support, the other hand is then brought from the seat of the wheelchair to the armrest. Pushing on both armrests, patient lifts body over the seat of the wheelchair. The transfer is then complete by lowering the buttocks onto the seat, reattaching the footrests, placing her feet on the footrests, and properly positioning herself.

Some patients are able to get sufficient height and momentum to seat themselves on the anterior part of the seat using the first push-up only. They can then reposition their hands and adjust their seating position.

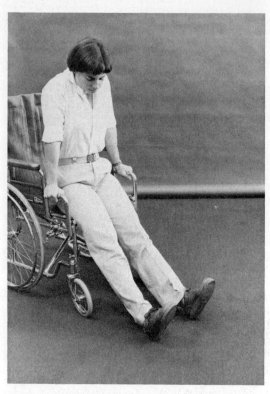

Pushing up to sit properly.

TURN AROUND METHOD TO FLOOR

The wheelchair is positioned with the casters forward and is locked. The footrests are removed or swung out of the way. The patient scoots to the front edge of the wheelchair seat. She then partially turns onto one hip.

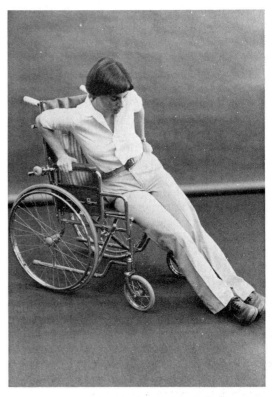

Initiating lowering from wheelchair to floor, turn around method.

She then moves the hand on the side to which she is turning behind her, grasping the opposite side armrest (right hand on left armrest). Her other hand is moved across the front of her body to grasp the opposite side armrest (left hand on right armrest).

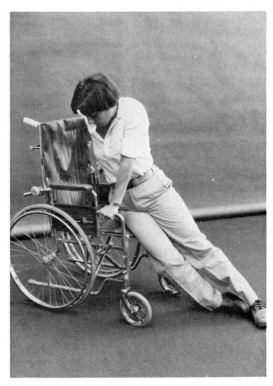

Adjusting hand position.

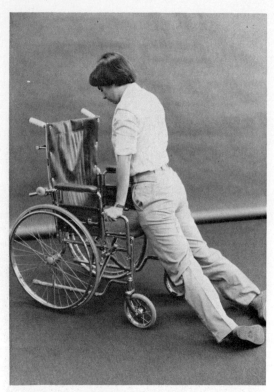

Pushing up to lift out of wheelchair.

As the patient extends her arms and depresses her shoulders, she completes the turn, facing the back of the wheelchair.

Once the turn has been completed, the patient lowers herself to the kneeling position. From the kneeling position she can move directly to the side-sitting position or the hands-knees position.

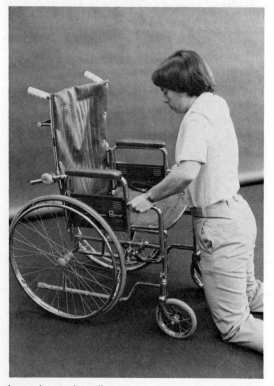

Lowering to kneeling.

TURN AROUND RETURN TO WHEELCHAIR

The wheelchair is positioned and locked with the casters turned forward. The footrests are removed or swung out of the way. The patient assumes the hands-knees position facing the wheelchair seat.

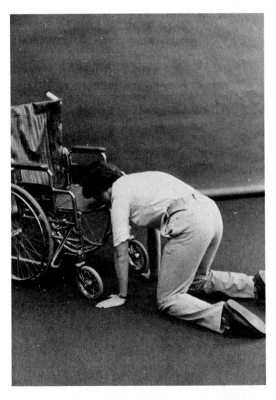

Starting position for return to wheelchair; turn around method.

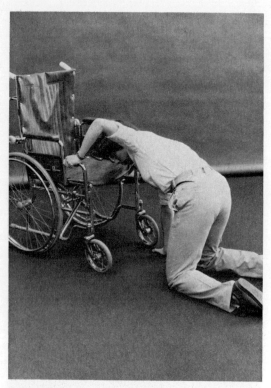

Preparing to attain kneeling.

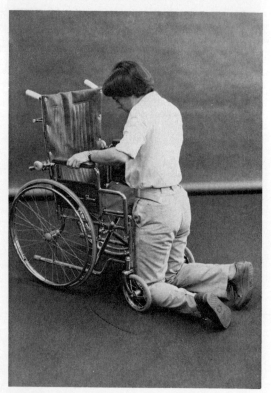

Kneeling; facing wheelchair.

The patient places one hand on the lower part of the armrest, or seat if the wheelchair does not have desk armrests. She then pushes to the kneeling position, placing the other hand on the top of the armrest as she attains the kneeling position. The hand on the seat or lower part of the armrest is then moved to the top of the armrest. Some patients may keep both hands on the lower part of the armrest as they push up.

Extending the arms and depressing the shoulders, the patient lifts herself.

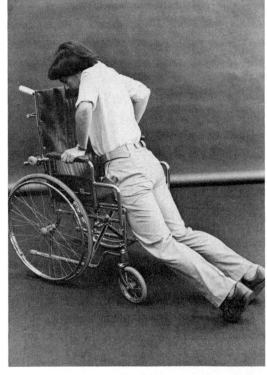

Pushing up to assist self into wheelchair.

The patient then initiates a turn as she lowers herself onto the seat of the wheelchair.

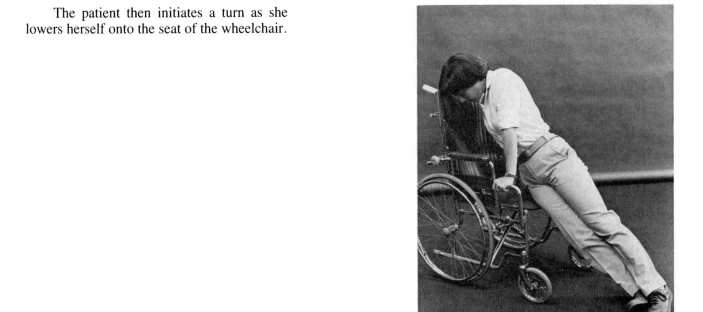

Pivoting onto side in wheelchair.

The hands are then repositioned onto the appropriate armrests. She can then complete the turn and properly position herself on the seat of the wheelchair. The footrests can then be replaced, and the patient's feet properly positioned.

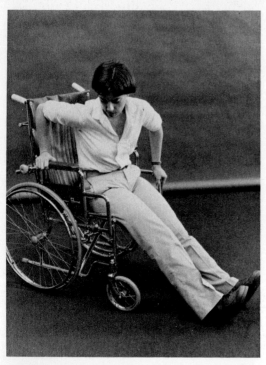

Adjusting sitting position.

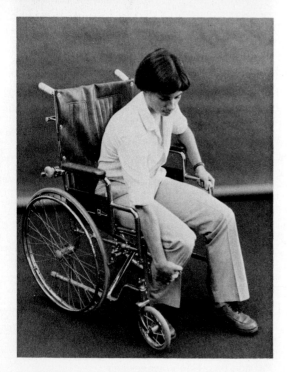

Positioning leg for transferring forward out of wheelchair.

FORWARD TO HANDS-KNEES

The wheelchair is positioned and locked with the caster wheels forward. The footrests are removed or swung out of the way. The patient scoots forward to the edge of the wheelchair seat and places her feet under her.

Grasping the lower portion of the armrests, the patient lowers herself to the kneeling position.

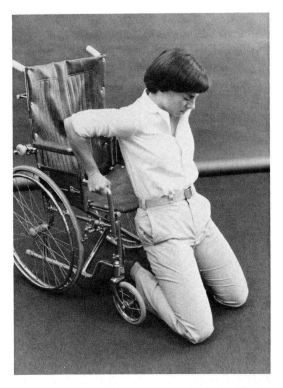

Lowering to kneeling.

As she bends forward, the patient places one hand on the floor. The other hand is then placed on the floor so that the patient is now in the hands-knees position.

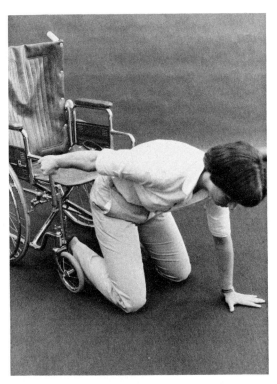

Lowering one hand to floor.

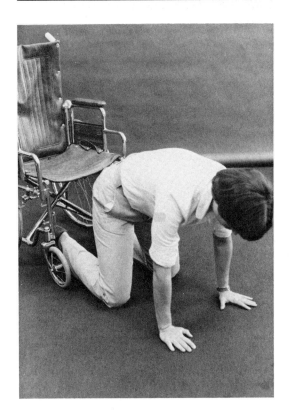

Hands-knees position.

9
AMBULATION WITH ASSISTIVE DEVICES

INTRODUCTION

Assistive devices are used to make safe ambulation possible. The three main indications for using assistive devices are (1) decreased ability to bear weight on the lower extremities resulting from structural damage of the skeletal system, (2) muscle weakness or paralysis of the trunk or lower extremities, and (3) poor balance in the upright posture. Assistive devices increase the base of support, allowing a redistribution of weight within the base of support, and a larger area within which the center of gravity can shift without losing balance.

When using assistive devices, the energy cost of ambulation can be very high. This, in addition to learning a new sequence of walking, can cause a patient to fatigue rapidly. In early training sessions, the patient will require greater concentration to learn the proper gait pattern. This use of the mind will prevent or interfere with the patient's ability to respond to other inputs, such as questions and normal conversation. The patient may stop walking in order to answer questions. Extraneous conversation with, and around, the patient should be avoided during initial training. However, later in training, such additional inputs can be used to test the degree to which the patient has learned the new gait pattern.

TIPS ON TEACHING

Instruction in a gait pattern often begins in the parallel bars because they provide maximum stability, and require the least amount of coordination by the patient. The patient can become accustomed to the upright posture and learn the sequence for gait in the relative safety of the parallel bars. The assistive device can be fitted while the patient stands in the parallel bars. This also allows the patient to practice standing or the sequence for gait while waiting for the therapist to adjust the assistive device to the proper height, providing an efficient use of treatment time. Readjustment of the fit of an assistive device may be necessary after a patient has become proficient in use of the assistive device.

Initial use of the assistive devices can be in, or alongside, the parallel bars. The patient has the reassurance that the stable parallel bars are readily available should the assistive device prove to be unstable at first. However, the patient may become too dependent on the parallel bars, so the therapist must progress the patient to ambulation away from the parallel bars as rapidly as possible.

The therapist should describe and demonstrate to the patient the proper use of the assistive device, and the appropriate gait sequence, before the patient begins amubulating. Generally, a demonstration is the primary method of instruction, and a verbal description reinforces the demonstration. Thus, the verbal description should be kept to a minimum. Observing other patients who are using assistive devices correctly can also be a useful method of instruction.

Once a patient is proficient on level surfaces, instruction in the use of stairs, curbs, ramps, and doors is given. The patient should be taught to ascend and descend stairs on the right-hand side because that is the usual method used in the United States. Instruction in sitting down and standing up when using armless chairs, low or soft sofas and chairs, toilets, and car seats is also necessary. In addition, patients must be taught how to protect themselves during a fall, and

NWB   non wt bearing
PWB   partial wt.
FWB   Full wt.

how to get up after a fall. Some patients may need the opportunity to walk with assistive devices on uneven surfaces, such as an unpaved sidewalk or parking lot, and to cross a street in the time allotted by one red light cycle. These circumstances are dictated by the patient's needs in order to function in the home or work setting.

The patient must be instructed to check the assistive device for safe condition for use. The wing nuts used on crutches often loosen with use. The rubber tips of assistive devices will not grip the floor properly if they become worn excessively, or dirt fills the grooves. The patient should also be warned to avoid small throw rugs that may slip or become entangled when the assistive device is placed on them. Wet or highly polished floors should also be avoided.

CHOOSING AN ASSISTIVE DEVICE

INTRODUCTION

A variety of assistive devices for gait is available. Some devices provide more stability and support than others. Some devices also require more coordination to use. As the patient's abilities increase, the patient may progress from a device that provides much stability and support to one that provides less stability and support. Other patients continue to use the same device throughout the entire time an assistive device is required. The following list of assistive devices is in order from most stable and supportive to least stable and supportive:

1. Parallel bars
2. Walker
3. Axillary crutches
4. Forearm (Lofstrand) crutches
5. Two canes
6. One cane

The following list of assistive devices is in order from those requiring the least patient coordination to those requiring the most patient coordination:

1. Parallel bars
2. Walker
3. Cane
4. Crutches

A special platform can be attached to walkers or crutches for patients who are unable to bear weight through their hand, wrist, or forearm, or who have poor grasp.

On some occasions one crutch may be used as an intermediate step between two crutches and one cane, or instead of one cane.

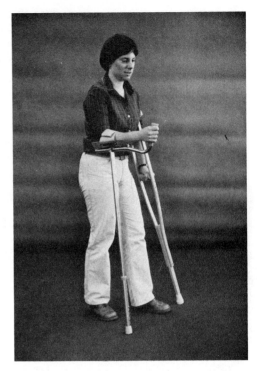

Platform crutch and axillary crutch.

When selecting an assistive device, the therapist must choose one that will provide the necessary support and that the patient can manipulate. Thus, the choice of an assistive device is based on the patient's stability, coordination, and disability. For example, a patient with a fractured leg who is to be nonweight bearing may use crutches if she has the stability and coordination necessary to use them. Another patient with the same fracture may require the use of a walker because of poor stability or coordination. Assistive devices come in several sizes—tall, standard, junior and child.

WALKERS

Walkers provide stability and are easy to use, but they are cumbersome. When possible, a collapsible walker should be used. A collapsible walker is easier to transport in a car, and can be placed out of the way in public places, such as movies and restaurants.

A special adaption of the walker is a hemi-walker. It has a handgrip attached to the center crossbar. Thus a patient with only one functional arm can use it for ambulation.

Walkers are also available with 2 or 4 wheels. Walkers with wheels should have a brake that is activated during weight bearing on the walker to insure stability.

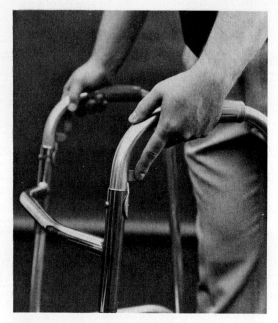

One type of collapsible walker.

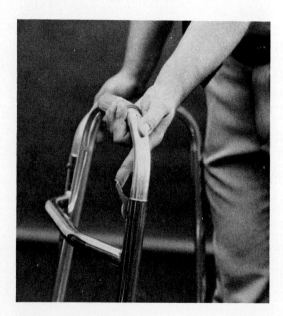

Walker partially collapsed.

AXILLARY AND FOREARM (LOFSTRAND) CRUTCHES

Axillary crutches are usually chosen for the patient who will need crutches for a relatively short period of time. Axillary crutches are easier to use than forearm crutches, but are also more restrictive. Forearm (Lofstrand)-crutches are recommended for patients who will need crutches permanently, or for long periods of time, and who have the stability, strength, and coordination to use them. Forearm crutches allow the patient greater maneuverability and are less wearing on the patient's clothing.

CANES

Several styles of canes are available. The standard is known as a J-line cane because of its shape. A common variation is the bent cane. The purpose of the bent cane is to have the weight bearing directly over the tip in contact with the floor. The grip is also varied in shape and texture to make grasp easier.

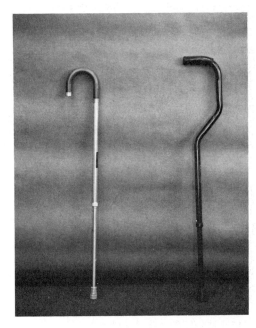

J-line cane (left) and bent cane (right).

Canes normally use in the hand of opposite side involved

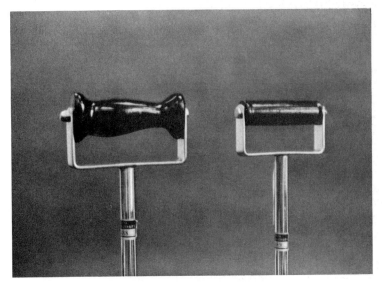

Variations of cane grips.

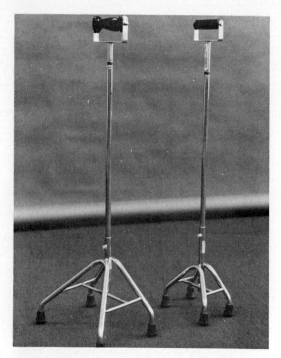

Large-base quad cane (left) and small-base quad cane (right).

A useful variation of the cane is the quad cane; so named because it has four feet. The quad cane is available in two basic sizes, large base and small base. A quad cane is stable by nature of its design. The patient may let go of the cane without concern that it will fall or slide to the floor as the standard canes do.

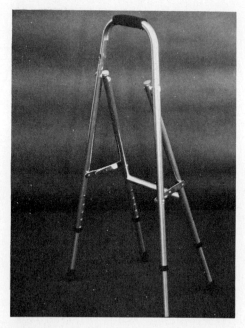

Walker-cane

A walker-cane has a larger base of support than a quad cane and requires less space for storage than a walker. A walker-cane is used in the same manner as a standard cane except for stairs.

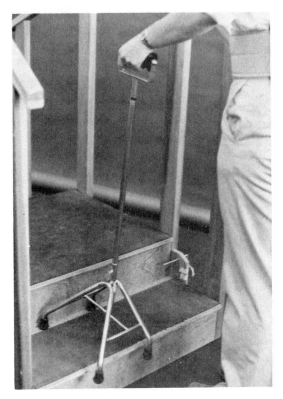

Improper fit of quad cane on a stair tread.

A disadvantage of the large base quad cane is the fact that it will not fit on a standard stair tread unless turned sideways.

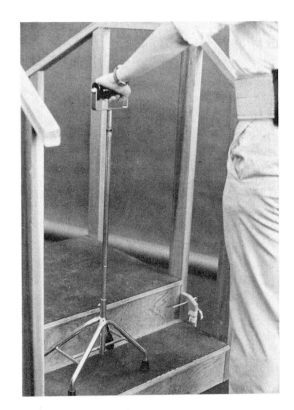

Correct use of quad cane on stair tread.

CHOOSING A GAIT PATTERN

The amount of weight bearing permitted depends upon the illness or injury involved. A gait pattern is determined by the amount of weight bearing permitted. Weight bearing may be varied form the extremes of no weight bearing to full weight bearing. The gait patterns commonly used to vary weight bearing loads, in ascending order from least weight reduction to most weight reduction; are

1. Four-point
2. Two-point
3. Three-point

The gait pattern used for muscle weakness or paralysis depends upon the severity of the condition. Gait patterns commonly used for such conditions are

1. Swing-to
2. Swing-through
3. Four-point
4. Three-point
5. Two-point

Gait patterns commonly used for balance, in ascending order from least support to greatest support, are

1. Two-point
2. Four-point

GETTING A PATIENT TO STANDING

In order to come to standing, the patient must be sitting on the edge of the chair or seat. With the patient on the edge of the chair, the patient's feet can be placed most directly underneath the body. Thus the patient's center of gravity can be brought over the base of support quickly as standing is assumed. The patient should place both feet close to the front edge of the chair. The feet may be placed together, or they may be one in front of the other in a short stride position.

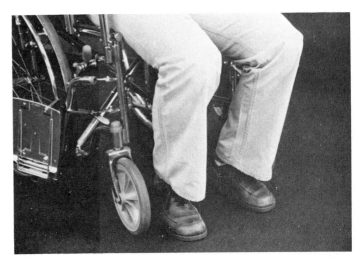

Feet together prior to standing.

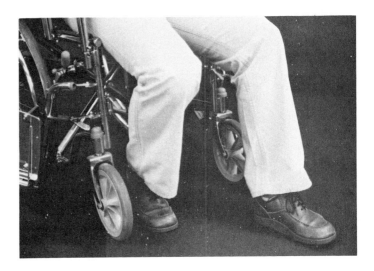

Feet in stride prior to standing.

Getting to the edge of the chair can be accomplished in a number of ways. The patient can perform sitting pushups, sliding forward each time a sitting pushup is performed, or the patient can unload one limb at a time, rotating forward each time a limb is unloaded. Unloading one limb at a time requires the patient to lean to one side, taking weight off the buttock on the other side. While the unloaded limb is not in contact with the seat, the patient can rotate that side forward. This is repeated, alternating sides. Illustrations of these maneuvers are found in chapter 8, pages 194 to 195.

The therapist can assist the patient with balance or lifting during these maneuvers. While standing in front of the patient, the therapist should place one arm around the shoulder on the side to which the patient is leaning. The therapist should not place his arm under the axilla as this interferes with the patient's arm movement and may also be uncomfortable. The therapist then places the other arm under the thigh or buttock to assist in lifting. Standing in front of the patient allows alternation of support from side to side as the patient shifts back and forth, without requiring extremes of movement by the therapist. Eventually the patient should reach the front edge of the chair.

When assuming the standing position, the patient must push in a directly downward direction with both arms and legs. If the patient pushes at an angle, the horizontal vector of the pushing force does not help the patient rise, and in fact may propel the patient horizontally, and thus off balance.

The patient must lean forward to shift her center of gravity over the feet, and then extend legs and trunk while pushing down slightly backward on the hands in order to come to standing.

The therapist usually stands slightly behind and to the side of the patient. If the patient is weak or has not stood for some time, the therapist may stand in front of the patient, as for an assisted standing pivot transfer, in order to provide assistance. The parallel bars would provide the most stability and safety in these situations.

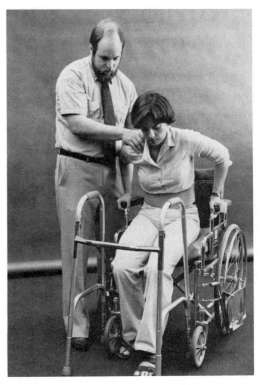

Therapist grasping gait belt; standing behind and slightly to side.

GUARDING

When ambulating a patient, a gait belt is used. A gait belt fits snugly around the patient's waist, and has handles for the therapist to hold. Holding onto a patient's belt may be uncomfortable for the patient as the narrow belt or belt buckle may bind. Clothing usually does not fit snugly enough to provide control, and clothing can tear, allowing the patient to fall.

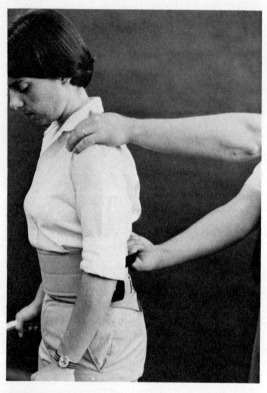

Grasping gait belt with supinated forearm and holding patient's shoulder.

The therapist stands in stride, behind and slightly to one side of the patient. The therapist grasps the gait belt with a supinated forearm because this provides a stronger grasp. The therapist's other hand is placed over the patients's shoulder, not on the arm where it may interfere with free motion needed to control an assistive device.

Note that the therapist is holding the patient's trunk, not the arm. As the patient's ability to ambulate improves, the therapist removes the hand on the patient's shoulder. As the patient walks, the therapist moves with the patient. The therapist's outside foot moves when the assistive device on that side is moved, and the therapist's inside foot is moved when the patient's foot is moved. This allows the therapist to move smoothly with the patient without kicking or tripping the patient, or interfering with the assistive device. During initial gait training, the therapist must stand close to the patient. As the patient improves, the therapist may stand farther from the patient.

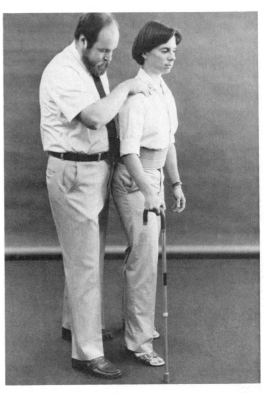

Proper guarding position during initial phase of gait training.

Initially, the therapist may stand on the patient's stronger side. This allows the therapist to pull the patient onto the stronger leg should the patient start to fall. Later, the therapist may stand on the patient's weaker side in order to encourage weight shifting and weight bearing on the weaker side.

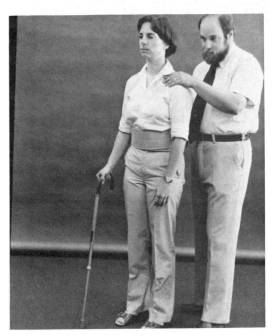

Proper guarding position during later phase of gait training.

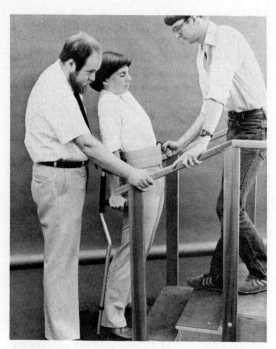

Preparing to ascend stairs with two assistants.

When guarding a patient on the stairs, the therapist positions himself below the patient. One of the therapist's hands grasps the gait belt, and the other hand holds the stair rail. Holding the stair rail provides the therapist with a point of stability. The therapist stands in stride, and as the patient and therapist progress up the stairs, the therapist always has his feet on different stair treads. Both feet are never on the same stair tread. This enables the therapist to shift his weight as the patient moves.

Occasionally a second person is needed to assist. This assistant also holds the gait belt and stair rail, and stands in stride on the stairs above the patient.

When ascending or descending stairs, the patient should be instructed to place the assistive device (crutches or cane) one half to two thirds of the way forward on the stair tread. The assistive devices should be placed to the sides to allow room for the patient's feet between the assistive devices. The stronger leg is advanced first when ascending stairs, as it must lift the body to the next higher step. the weaker leg and assistive device follow when moving up the stairs, either at the same time or separately. When descending, the weaker leg and assistive device are moved to the next lower step first, either together or separately with the assistive device moving first. The stronger leg is used to lower the body to the step, and then the stronger leg is brought down to the same step.

Maneuvering through doors requires short steps and sharp turns by the patient. The therapist's position for guarding during these maneuvers is the same position as for guarding during regular ambulation with walkers, crutches, and canes. Realizing that shorter steps and abrupt turns may be required, the therapist should be prepared to turn and move quickly, avoiding interference with the patient's freedom of movement, or the arc of movement of the door.

In the following sections on ambulation through doorways with walkers and crutches, text and photographs depict independent ambulation. In this way a therapist did not obscure the desired views in the photographs. Guarded ambulation through doorways with walkers, crutches, and canes would be performed in the same sequence, with the therapist guarding in the usual manner, and assisting with the door as needed.

USING ASSISTIVE DEVICES

WALKERS

FITTING

To measure a walker for the proper height, the patient stands in the walker with the crossbar in front. The top of the handgrip should be approximately at the level of the patient's ulnar styloid process when her arm is relaxed at her side. When the patient grasps the handgrip, the shoulders should be level and relaxed, and the elbow flexed to 20° to 30°.

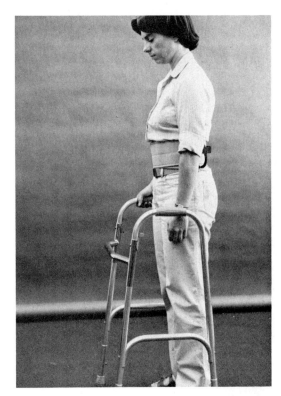

Measuring height of walker.

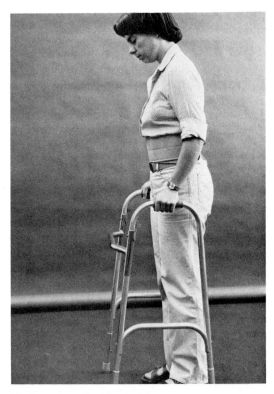

Walker correctly adjusted for use.

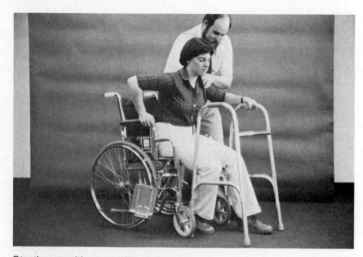

Starting position; coming to standing.

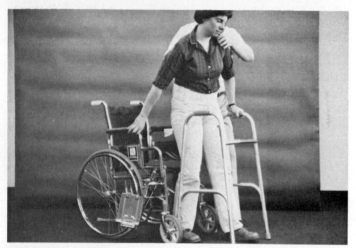

Pushing to standing.

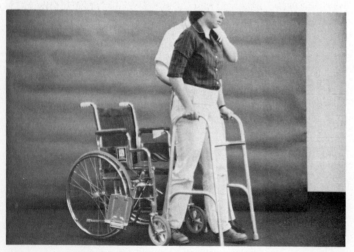

Ready to ambulate.

IN AND OUT OF WHEELCHAIR

Two methods of getting in and out of a wheelchair will be described. In both methods the wheelchair is positioned, locked, and the footrests are removed or swung out of the way. The patient moves to the front edge of the wheelchair seat and places her feet directly underneath.

In the first method, the feet are in stride with the stronger foot forward. The hand on the stronger side grasps and pushes down on the handgrip of the walker. This insures that the patient is moving into her strength. The patient pushes to standing using one handgrip of the walker and one armrest of the wheelchair. The patient's other hand is then placed on the walker handgrip. The therapist stands behind and to one side of the patient.

The disadvantage of this method is that the walker may tip sideways. The force exerted on the walker must be exerted downward to avoid tipping.

To sit, the patient walks to the wheelchair, turns toward her stronger side, and walks backward until the front edge of the wheelchair seat is felt against the back of the legs. The feet are in stride, with the stronger leg back. The patient reaches backward for the armrest with the arm on the stronger side first. The patient slowly lowers herself to sitting. The other hand is moved to the armrest, and the patient adjusts her sitting position. The therapist moves as the patient moves, maintaining his position behind and to the side of the patient.

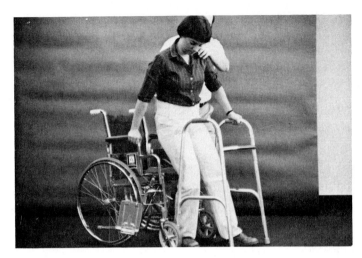

Reaching back to armrest and lowering to seat.

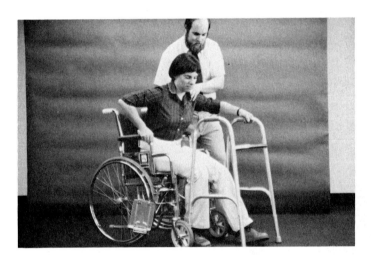

Sitting down.

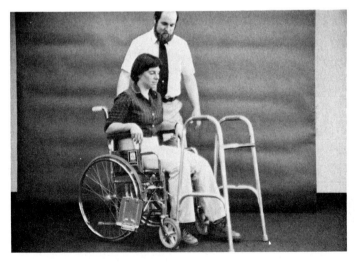

Readjusting position in wheelchair.

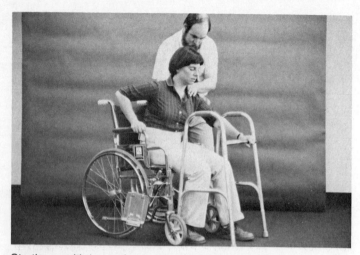

Starting position; coming to standing using crossbar.

In the second method, the wheelchair and patient are prepared as in the first method. The patient places the hand of the stronger side on the crossbar of the walker. The other hand is placed on the armrest. The feet are placed in stride, and the stronger foot forward. The patient pushes to standing, and then moves her hand from the armrest to the handgrip of the walker. The hand on the crossbar of the walker is then moved to the handgrip of the walker.

This method is easier for some patients. However, the force on the crossbar must be directed downward, or the walker will tilt or slide.

Many patients have less trouble with the walker tipping when using this method. This method enables the patient to use the arm on the walker efficiently when pushing directly downward on the walker.

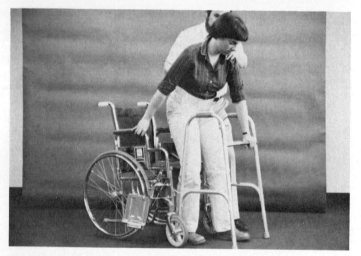

Standing with primary weight bearing on left extremities.

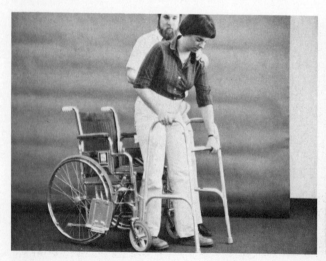

Repositioned right hand.

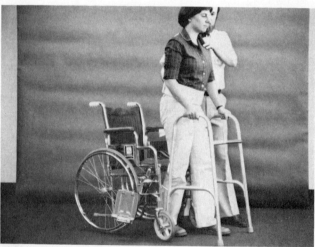

Repositioned left hand; ready to ambulate.

To sit, the patient reverses the process. With the hand of the weaker side on the crossbar, the patient places the hand of the stronger side on the wheelchair armrest. The feet are in stride, with the stronger leg back. The patient slowly lowers herself to sitting.

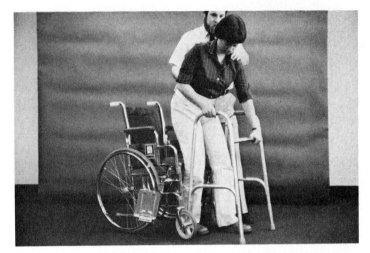

Positioning hand prior to sitting.

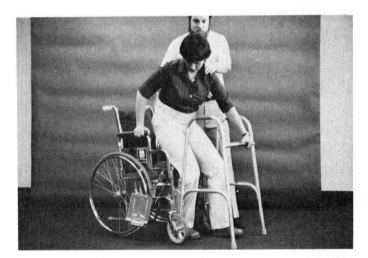

Holding armrest; lowering to seat.

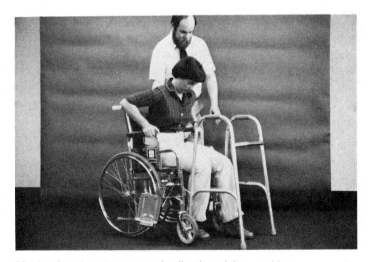

Moving hand to armrest and adjusting sitting position.

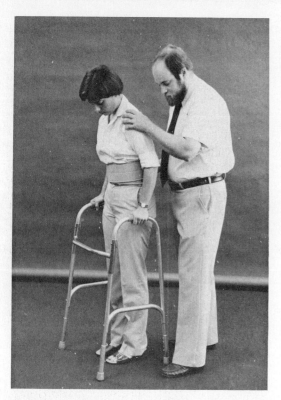

Starting position for walker; three-point gait pattern.

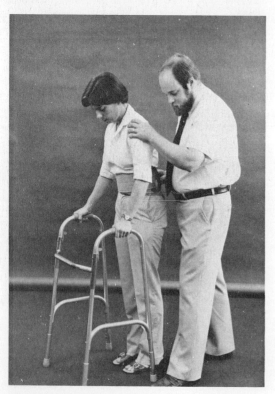

Patient advances walker.

AMBULATION WITH THREE-POINT GAIT PATTERN

To ambulate using the three-point gait pattern, the patient stands in the middle of the walker. The walker is lifted and advanced forward. All four legs must be lifted from the ground, and all four legs must contact the floor at one time when the walker is lowered.

As the patient moves the walker, the therapist advances his left, outside leg.

The patient advances her weaker leg, thus moving into the strength and stability of the walker.

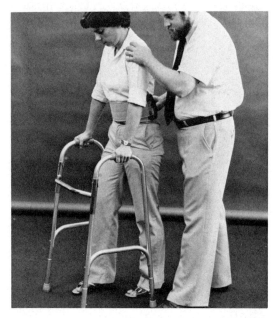

Patient advances weaker leg.

The patient bears weight through her arms as she advances her stronger leg. She may step to, or slightly beyond, her other foot. Equal step lengths should be encouraged. The therapist advances his right, or inside, leg in order to move with the patient.

The total sequence is repeated for continued progression.

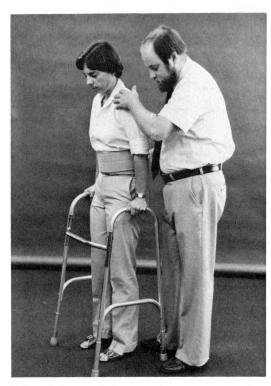

Patient advances stronger leg.

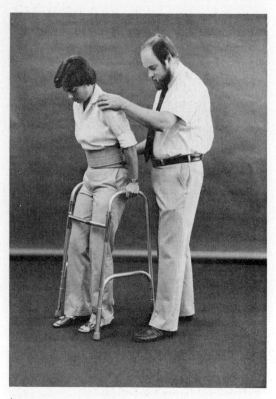

Improper use; stepping beyond crossbar.

The patient should not step beyond the crossbar because this does not allow her to stand erect, which is necessary to advance the walker for the next step.

AMBULATION WITH SWING-TO GAIT PATTERN

The second gait pattern that may be used with the walker is the swing-to gait pattern. This pattern may be used when both lower extremities are weak and are involved to approximately the same degree.

The patient stands in the walker and the therapist assumes the guarding position.

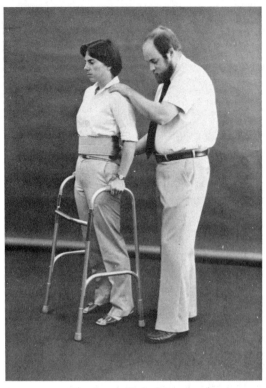

Starting position for walker; swing-to gait pattern.

The walker is advanced, and the therapist advances his outside leg.

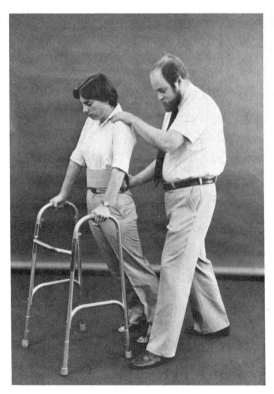

Patient advances walker.

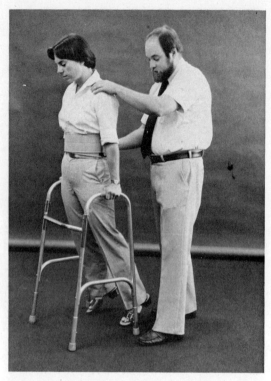

Patient lifts herself and swings forward.

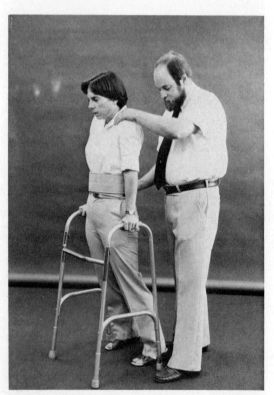

Patient lowers herself.

The patient extends her arms and depresses her shoulders while pushing down on the handgrips of the walker in order to lift her body. The patient can then let her body swing forward, or swing to, the walker. The therapist moves his inside leg as the patient swings forward.

The patient lowers herself at the end of the swing and bears weight on her legs. The sequence is repeated for continued progression.

AMBULATION ON STAIRS

Although it is not the most stable device on stairs, the walker can be used when ambulating on the stairs. The patient should turn the walker sideways so the crossbar is next to the patient. One hand is placed on the forwardmost handgrip of the walker and the other hand grasps the stair rail.

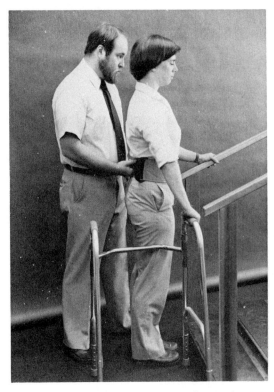

Starting position for walker, ascending stairs.

The patient places the two forwardmost legs of the walker on the upper stair.

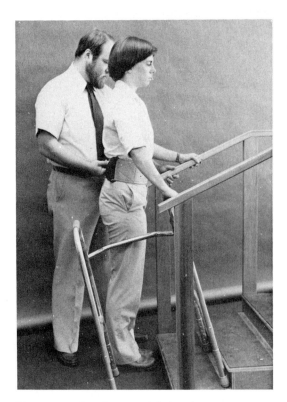

Placement of walker on stair treads.

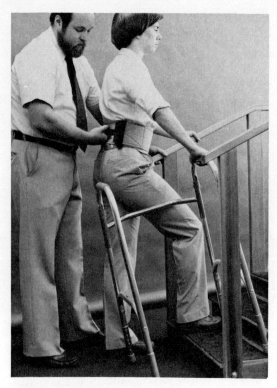

Patient advances stronger leg.

The patient then advances her stronger leg onto the stair. The stronger leg leads because it must lift the patient onto the higher stair. The therapist stands in stride behind the patient. One hand grasps the gait belt and the other hand grasps the stair rail.

The weaker leg is advanced to the same stair as the stronger leg.

The sequence is repeated for continued progression.

The same sequence can be used to ascend a curb, provided someone or something can substitute for the stair rail. An alternative method is to place the walker on the sidewalk and use the walker in the normal manner.

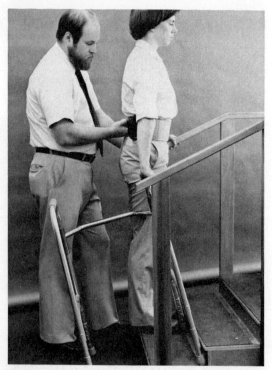

Patient advances weaker leg to same stair as stronger leg.

To descend stairs, the walker is again turned sideways. The two forwardmost legs of the walker are placed on the lower stair, and the patient grasps the rear handgrip of the walker with one hand and the stair rail with the other hand. The therapist stands in stride in front of the patient, grasping the gait belt with one hand and the stair rail with the other hand.

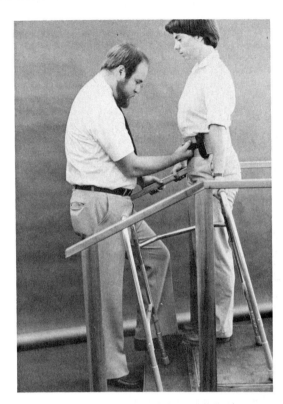

Starting position for walker, descending stairs.

The patient lowers the weaker leg to the lower stair. The stronger leg is then brought to the same stair as the weaker leg.

The same sequence is repeated for continued progression.

The same sequence may be used to descend a curb, provided the patient has someone or something to substitute for the stair rail. An alternative is to place the walker on the street in front of the patient. The walker is then used in the normal manner.

Special stair climbing walkers are available. These walkers have handgrips extending backwards from the back uprights.

When ascending stairs, the walker is turned around and placed behind the patient. The two legs with the handgrips are placed on the first stair while the other two legs remain on the floor. The extended handgrips are used by the patient.

When descending stairs, the walker is placed in the normal position. The legs without extended handgrips are in front, and are placed on the lower stair, while the legs with the extended handgrips remain on the upper stair.

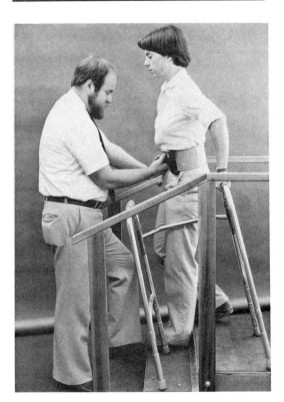

Weaker leg is lowered first.

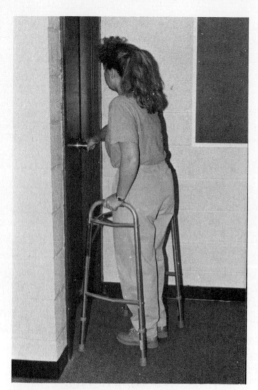

Starting position to open door opening away from patient.

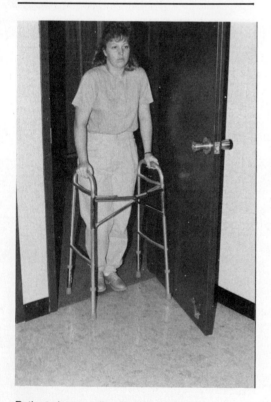

Patient places walker feet as a door stop.

AMBULATION THROUGH DOORWAYS

A variety of doors may necessitate teaching a variety of methods and modifications.

Doors Open Away from Patient—With Automatic Door Closer The patient approaches the opening edge of the door, and either faces the door directly, or turns sideways to the door with back towards the hinged edge of the door. The patient weight shifts to the side of the walker away from the hand that is to be used on the doorknob. The unweighted hand is then placed on the doorknob. Preferably, weight is shifted to the side away from the doorknob, and the hand closest to the doorknob can then be used to open the door.

Using a quick push, the door is open wider than necessary for the patient to move through the doorway. The wider opening of the door is necessitated by the fact that the door will start to close automatically until its closing is blocked by the walker. The hand on the doorknob is quickly returned to the walker which is placed in the path of the closing door. The feet on the side of the walker closest to the door are placed on the floor as a doorstop, as close to the opening edge as possible.

Using the walker feet as a doorstop, the patient steps into the doorway, past the opening edge of the door. Several small movements of the walker may be required as the patient steps through the doorway. At all times while the patient is moving through the doorway, the walker must remain in a position to act as a doorstop until the door will not strike the patient as it closes.

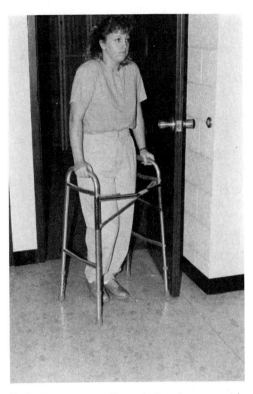

Patient progresses through the doorway, using walker feet as doorstop.

After determining that the arc of the closing door will not strike the patient, the patient and walker complete passage through the doorway, allowing the door to close automatically.

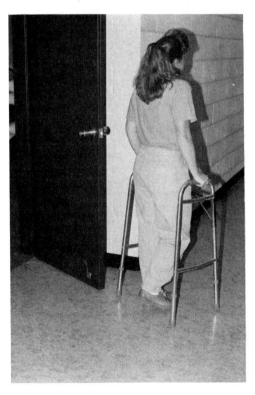

Patient completes passage through the doorway.

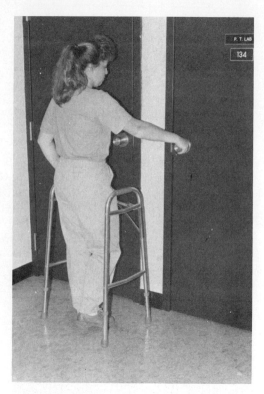

Starting position to open door swinging toward patient.

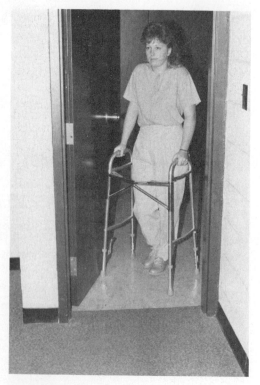

Patient opens door.

Door Opens Toward Patient—With Automatic Door Closer The patient approaches the opening edge of the door, standing outside the arc through which the opening door will move. The patient weight shifts to the side of the walker away from the hand that will be placed on the doorknob. The unweighted hand is then placed on the doorknob. Preferably, weight is shifted to the side away from the doorknob, and the hand closest to the doorknob can then be used to open the door.

Using a quick pulling motion, the door is pulled open past the patient, wider than is necessary for the patient to move through the doorway. The wider opening of the door is necessitated by the fact that the door will start to close automatically until its closing is blocked by the walker. The hand on the doorknob is quickly returned to walker, and the walker is placed in the path of the closing door. The feet on the side of the walker closest to the door are placed on the floor as a doorstop, as close to the opening edge as possible.

While maintaining the walker feet as a doorstop between the door and the patient, the patient steps into the doorway. Progressing through the doorway requires that the walker feet used as a doorstop are moved short distances and replaced on the ground quickly. This is necessary to prevent the automatic door closer from causing the door to hit the patient.

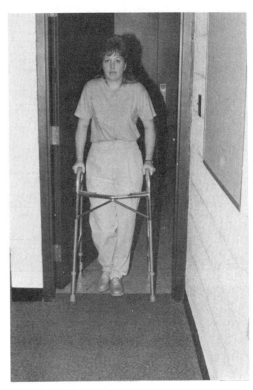

Patient progresses through the doorway, using walker feet as doorstop.

Once the patient and walker have completed passage through the doorway, the door closes.

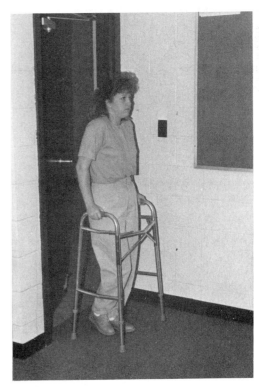

Patient completes passage through the doorway.

Without Automatic Door Closer When the door does not have an automatic closer, the initial rapid movement to place the walker feet on the ground as a doorstop is not necessary. The extra wide opening of the door is also not necessary. Because the door will not close automatically, the patient must turn to close the door.

AXILLARY CRUTCHES

FITTING

Axillary crutches are fitted with the patient standing. The crutches are positioned so the crutch tip rests on the floor approximately 6 inches away from the toes at 45° angle. The therapist should be able to put two or three fingers between the patient's axillae and the tops of the crutches. If a pad is to be used on the crutch top, it should be in place during the fitting.

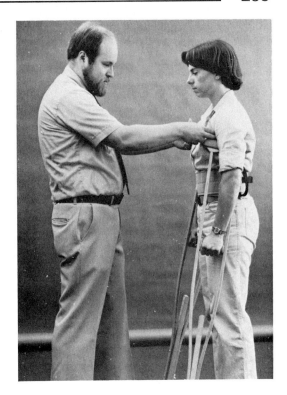

Checking fit of axillary crutches.

The handgrip height is adjusted to the level of the ulnar styloid process when the arm is relaxed at the patient's side. This will provide 20° to 30° of elbow flexion when holding the handgrip.

When ambulating with crutches, the lift is provided by shoulder depression and elbow extension. The patient must also adduct her arms to keep the crutches in place in the axillae. The patient must not rest on the top of the crutches because this will injure the nerves and block the blood vessels in the axillae, producing pain and tingling in the arms and hands. The result can be muscle weakness and possible paralysis.

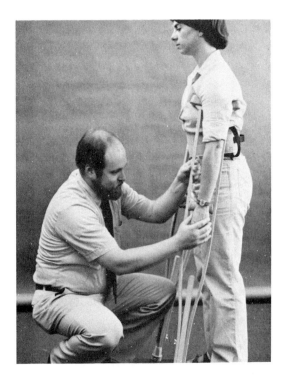

Measuring height of handgrips, axillary crutches.

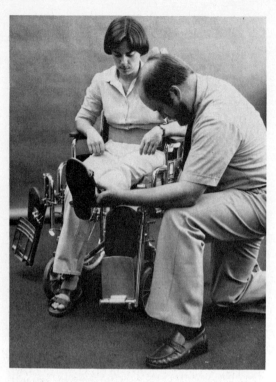

Removing legrest while supporting patient's leg.

IN AND OUT OF WHEELCHAIR

Before coming to standing, the wheelchair must be properly positioned and locked. The stronger leg is placed on the floor, and the footrest on that side of the wheelchair is removed or swung out of the way.

If the patient is unable to bend her knee, an elevating legrest is used to support the leg during sitting. The legrest must be removed or pivoted to the side before the patient stands in order to provide room for maneuvering. The crutches must be placed close at hand before the patient starts scooting forward.

The therapist supports the involved leg with one hand, and removes the legrest with the other hand.

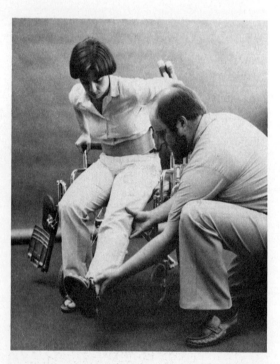

Lowering patient's leg; patient on front edge of seat.

The patient then scoots to the front edge of the seat of the wheelchair.

If the patient can tolerate, the involved leg is lowered to the floor before the patient attempts to stand. If not, the leg is lowered as the patient stands.

Using the handgrips, the patient grasps both crutches with the hand of the stronger side. The patient pushes to standing using the crutches on the stronger side and the armrest of the wheelchair on the other side. The therapist holds the patient by grasping the gait belt and lowering the involved extremity if necessary. If the patient needs more assistance, an assistant lowers the leg while the therapist guards the patient on the stronger side by grasping the gait belt and holding onto the patient's shoulder.

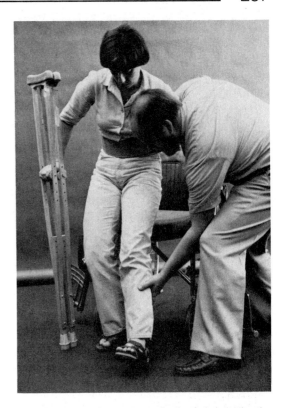

Pushing to standing; therapist lowering patient's leg.

Once the standing position is attained and the weight is being borne on the stronger side, the patient reaches across for a crutch.

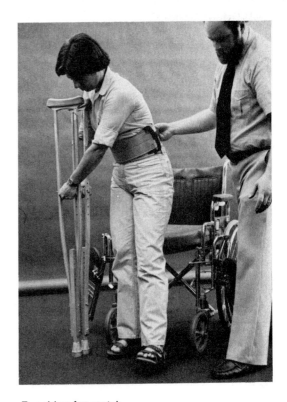

Reaching for crutch.

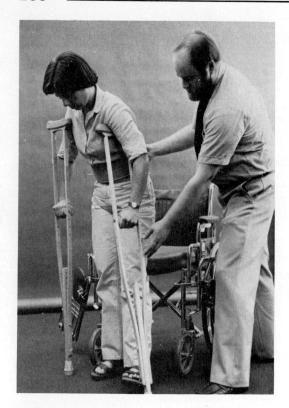

Placing crutch correctly.

The crutch is properly positioned in the axilla.

The other crutch is then properly positioned in the axilla.

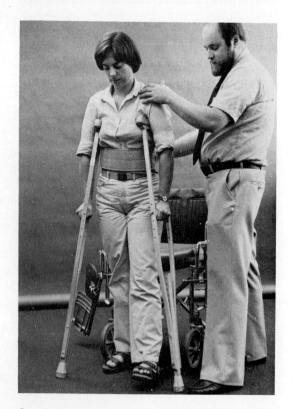

Crutches in place; ready for ambulation.

To sit, the patient walks toward the wheelchair, turns toward her stronger side, and backs up until the front edge of the wheelchair seat is felt against the back of the legs. The therapist positions himself on the involved side so that he is in a position to maneuver the patient's involved leg.

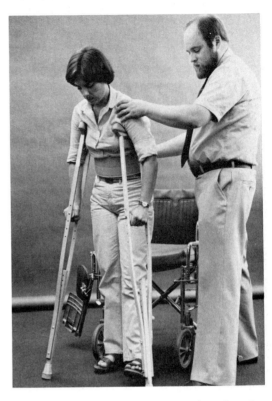

Walking backward to wheelchair; edge of seat felt behind knees.

The crutch on the patient's stronger side is removed from the axilla and held by the handgrip only.

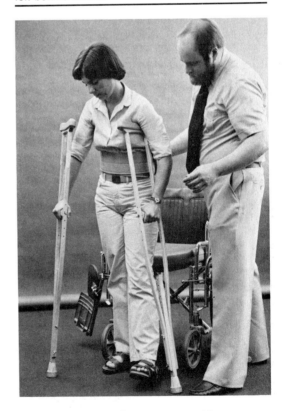

Re-positioning crutch on stronger side.

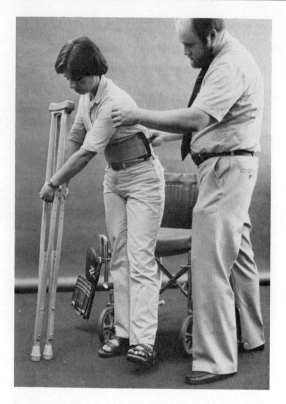

Placing other crutch on stronger side.

The other crutch is removed from the axilla and both crutches are held by the handgrips on the patient's stronger side

With the therapist holding the gait belt and assisting the involved leg if necessary, the patient reaches for the wheelchair armrest.

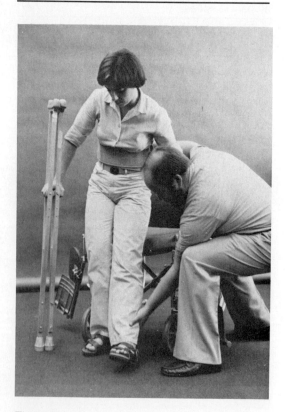

Therapist preparing to raise weaker leg as patient sits.

As the patient lowers herself to sitting, the therapist may need to elevate the patient's leg.

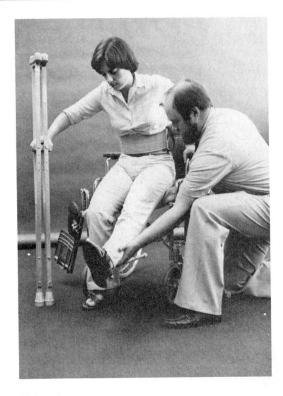

Sitting down.

The patient's leg is then placed in the appropriate position on the elevating legrest. The crutches are placed to the side, and the patient can adjust her position in the wheelchair.

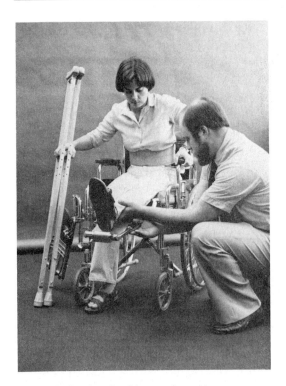

Repositioning involved leg on legrest.

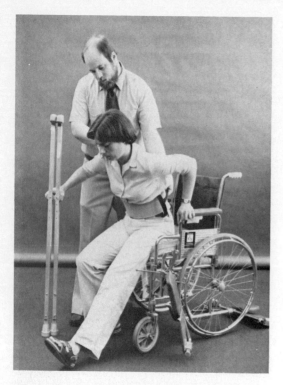

Patient can control involved let; placing it on floor ahead of stronger leg.

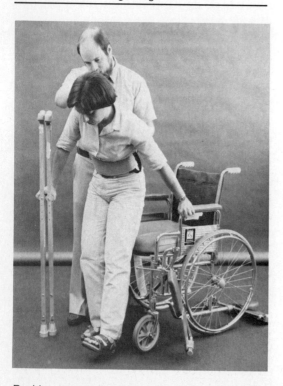

Pushing to standing; primary weight bearing on stronger limb.

If the patient can control her involved leg, the therapist will assist the patient to standing from the patient's stronger side. This allows the therapist to help the patient shift her weight and maintain her balance on the stronger leg. The crutches are placed together on the stronger side, and the patient grasps both by the handgrips only. The patient's other hand is on the armrest of the wheelchair. This allows the patient to move into her strength. The patient can then push to standing.

The crutches are positioned under the axillae one at a time.

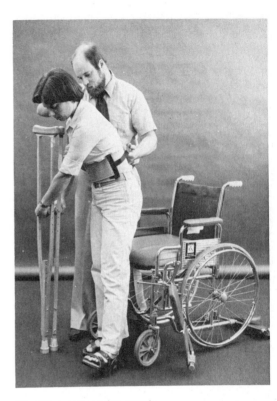

Reaching across for crutch.

The therapist is positioned behind and slightly to the side of the patient, and the patient is ready to ambulate.

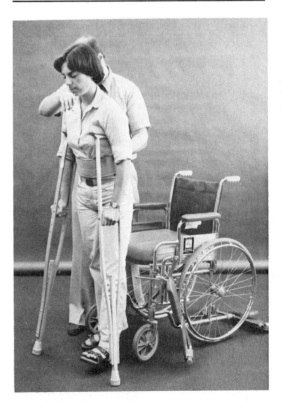

Properly placing crutches for ambulation.

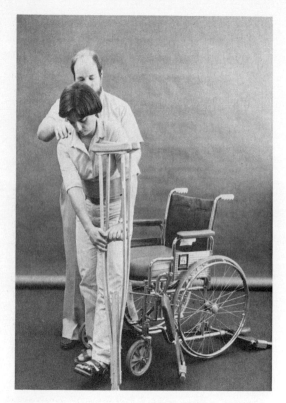

Placing both crutches in hand on involved side.

When the patient can control her involved leg, the therapist assists the patient to sitting from the patient's stronger side. The patient positions the involved leg slightly forward in order to sit. The crutches are placed together on the involved side and held by the handgrips only. The patient reaches for the armrest of the wheelchair with her stronger arm, allowing her to move into her strength.

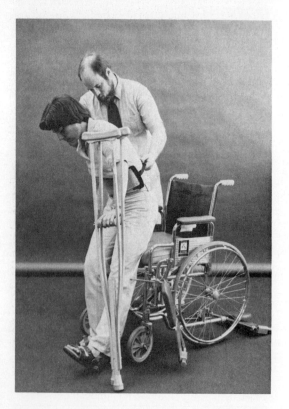

Reaching back for armrest and lowering to seat.

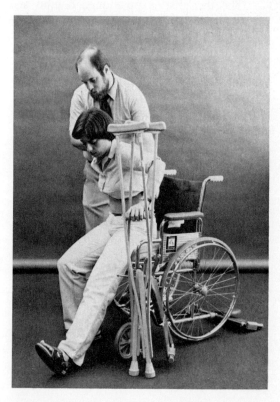

Completing assumption of sitting position.

AMBULATION WITH THREE-POINT GAIT PATTERN

A three-point gait pattern is used when one leg is involved. In the three-point gait pattern, the crutches moving together as a unit are considered one point. Each foot moves separately, and thus each is considered a point. This is the reason for the name three-point gait pattern.

The involved leg may be non-weight bearing, partial weight bearing, or full weight bearing, depending upon the patient's condition.

In the starting position, the crutches are placed parallel, in the same position used for measuring crutch fit. The feet are together. The therapist stands behind and slightly to the side of the patient.

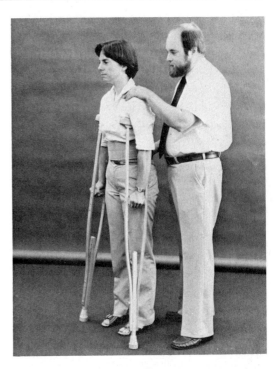

Starting position for axillary crutches; three-point gait pattern.

To ambulate, both crutches are advanced the same amount at the same time. The therapist advances his outside foot.

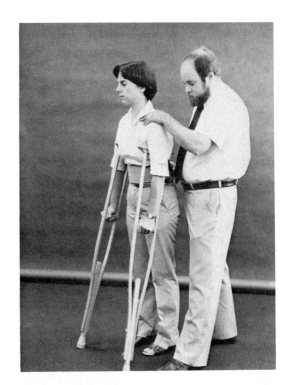

Patient advances both crutches.

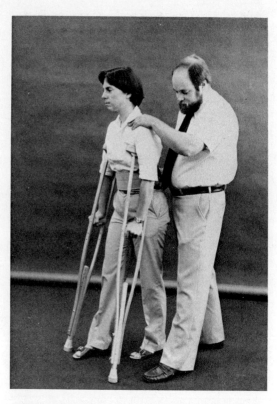

Patient steps to crutch with involved leg.

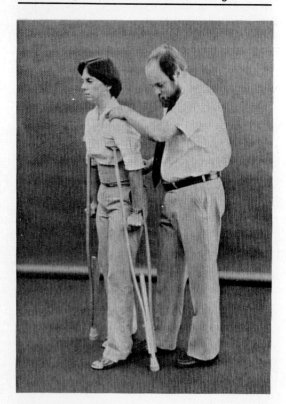

Patient steps through crutches with stronger leg.

The patient advances her weaker leg so the toes are even with the crutch tips. As the patient improves, she may move the crutches and involved leg at the same time. This allows for a faster pace of gait.

Using her arms to support her body weight, the patient advances her stronger foot beyond the crutches. Initially, the patient may "step to" her weaker leg, rather than "step through." Stepping through is the normal gait pattern, and should be encouraged. The therapist advances her inside leg as the patient moves her stronger leg.

The sequence is repeated for continued progression.

AMBULATION WITH FOUR-POINT GAIT PATTERN

With a four-point gait pattern, each crutch and each foot is moved separately, hence the name of the pattern. The four-point gait pattern is used when the patient has pain or weakness in both lower extremities of approximately the same severity, or needs assistance for balance when walking.

The starting position is the same as for a three-point pattern.

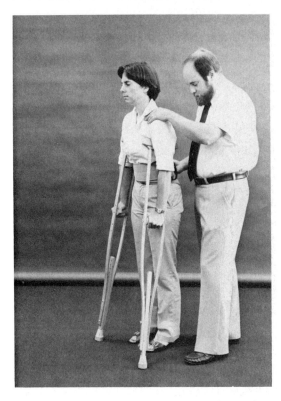

Starting position for axillary crutches; four-point gait pattern.

To ambulate, the patient advances one crutch; in this case, the left crutch. The therapist advances his outside foot.

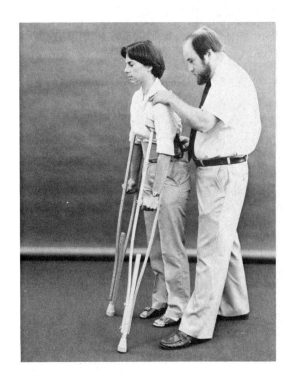

Patient advances left crutch.

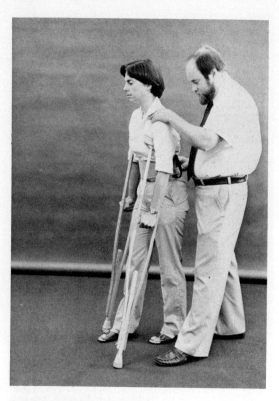

Patient advances right foot.

The patient then advances her opposite (in this example her right) leg to a point even with the tip of the left crutch.

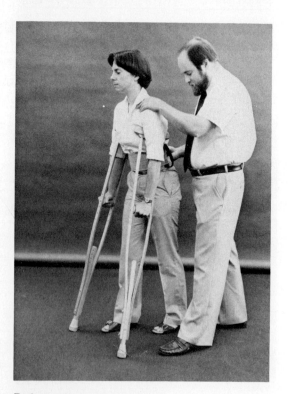

Patient advances right crutch.

The patient then advances the other (in the example her right) crutch slightly beyond the left crutch.

Finally, the patient advances her other (in this case her left) foot to a point even with the tip of her right crutch. The therapist advances his inside, or right, foot.

The sequence is repeated for continued progression.

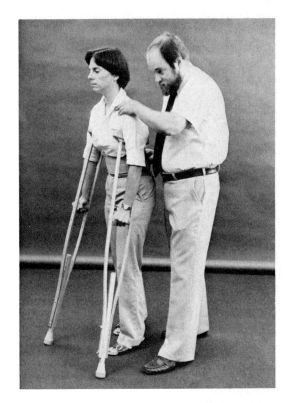

Patient advances left foot.

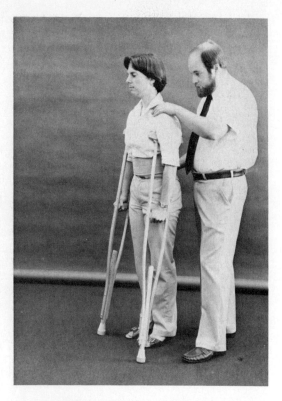

Starting position for axillary crutches; two-point gait pattern.

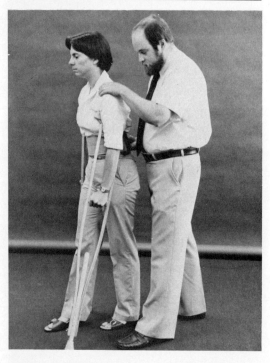

Patient advances left crutch and right foot at the same time.

AMBULATION WITH TWO-POINT GAIT PATTERN

The two-point gait pattern is considered a progression from the four-point gait pattern. A faster pace of ambulation is achieved. As patients become proficient with a four-point gait pattern, they may automatically begin using a two-point gait pattern.

The starting position is the same as for the three-point gait pattern.

The patient advances one crutch and the opposite foot together, placing the toes even with the tip of the crutch. In this example, the left crutch and right foot have been advanced together. The therapist moves his outside, or left, foot at this time.

The patient then advances her remaining (right) crutch and (left) foot together as the other point. This crutch and foot are advanced beyond the other crutch and foot in a normal stride length. The therapist moves his inside (right) foot at this time.

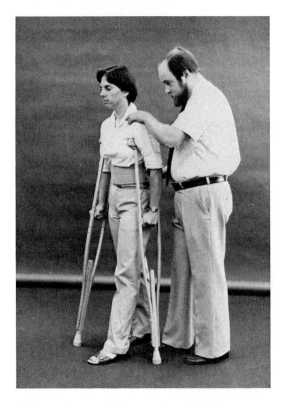

Patient advances right crutch and left foot at the same time.

FALLING

If a patient starts to fall, the therapist must decide to prevent the fall or to control the fall in a manner that will prevent injury to the patient or himself. In the method illustrated below, the therapist prevents a fall by shifting his weight onto his back foot and pulling the patient into him. This brings the patient into the therapist's base support. This is the reason for always guarding the patient from behind and slightly to the side, and standing in a stride. The patient is assisted to regain the starting position of the desired gait pattern, and progress can continue.

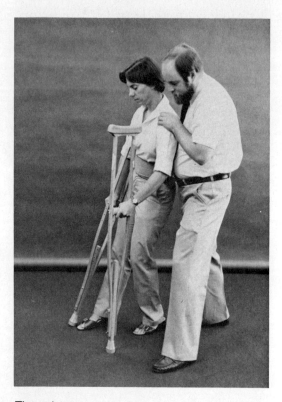

Therapist prevents a fall.

If the therapist cannot prevent the fall, he controls the fall. The patient is instructed to let the crutches fall to the side in order to avoid injury from landing on them. The therapist steps forward from his stride position to widen the base of support as he slows the patient's fall.

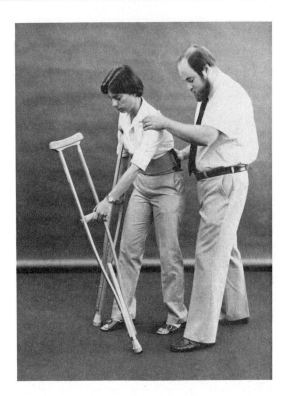

Therapist controls a fall.

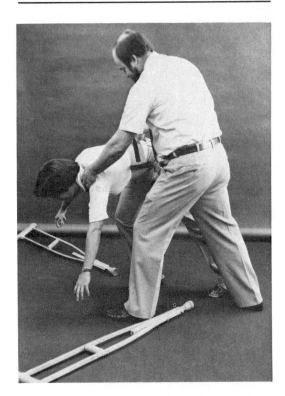

Patient lets crutches fall to side; prepares to catch herself.

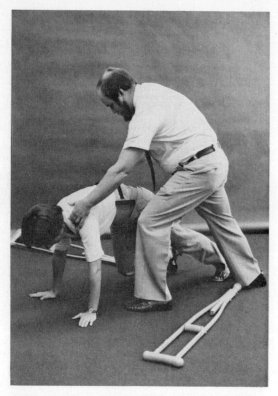

Therapist lowers patient; controlling rate of fall.

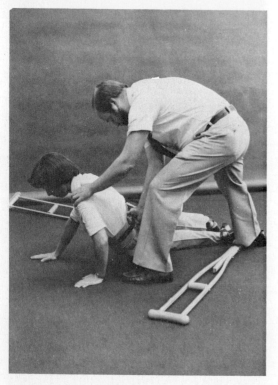

Patient turns onto stronger side.

The patient catches herself on her outstretched hands, making sure that the elbows bend to absorb the impact. If this is not done, injury to the patient's arms may occur. The therapist continues to lower the patient to the floor slowly, and the patient finishes the fall by turning onto the side of the strong leg. She is then in a position to initiate getting up from the floor.

The therapist must be alert to the patient's movements at all times, and act quickly to prevent or control a fall. This requires proper position and attention at all times.

AMBULATION ON STAIRS

Training to use the stairs is begun by having the patient use the stair rail and the crutch or crutches under the other arm. As illustrated, there are three ways the patient can hold the crutches in order to have them both in her possession when she reaches the top of the stairs. The most practical method is to place the crutches together under one arm. Whether two crutches and a stair rail, one crutch and a stair rail, or two crutches without a stair rail are used, the sequence of leg and assistive device movements is the same.

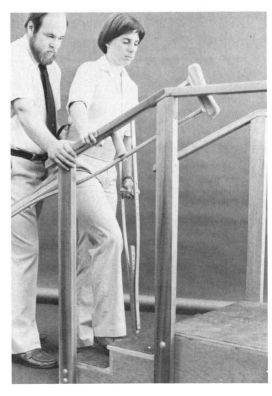

Holding crutch in hand grasping stair rail.

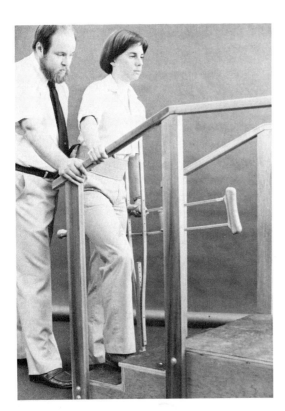

Holding crutch in hand opposite stair rail.

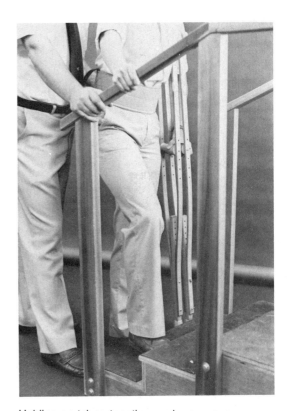

Holding crutches together under one arm.

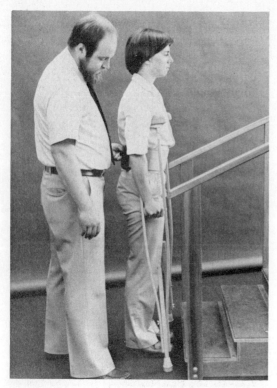

Starting position to ascend stairs; using both crutches.

The starting position to ascend stairs using both crutches is facing the stairs with both the crutches and the patient's feet parallel at the base of the first step. The therapist is behind the patient, grasping the gait belt.

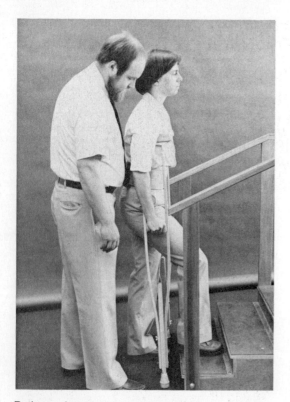

Patient advances stronger leg first.

The patient's stronger foot is placed on the stair while the body weight is supported by the arms.

The stronger leg is used to raise the body to the higher stair, and the crutches and weaker leg are advanced to the same stair. The therapist, standing behind the patient in stride, grasps the gait belt and stair rail. This sequence is repeated to ascend the entire flight of stairs, and may be used to ascend a curb.

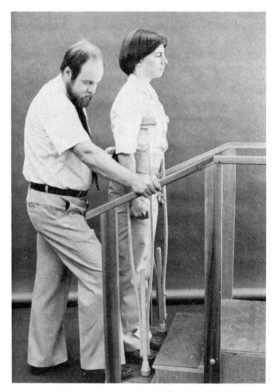

Involved leg and crutch are advanced to same stair.

In order to descend the stairs, the therapist stands in stride on the stairs, facing the patient as she approaches the stairs. The patient places both crutches and feet parallel to the first stair.

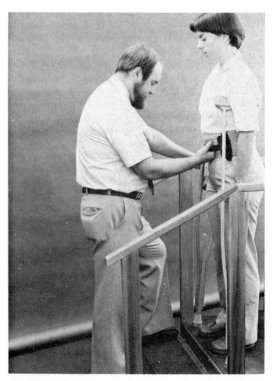

Starting position to descend stairs; using both crutches.

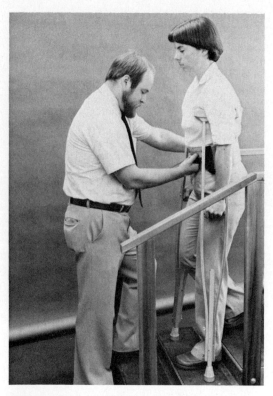

Patient lowers involved leg and crutches.

Using the stronger leg to lower the body weight, the crutches and weaker leg are lowered to the next lower stair. The crutches are placed two thirds of the distance from the back edge of the stair, and must be widely enough spaced to allow room for the patient.

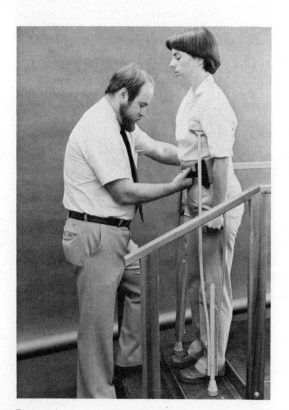

Patient lowers stronger leg to same stair.

With the body weight supported by the arms, the stronger leg is lowered to the same stair. The therapist moves backward down the stairs while grasping the gait belt and stair rail. He always maintains a stride stance while moving to provide room for the patient to descend to the next step.

The sequence is repeated in order to descend the full flight of stairs, and it may be used to descend a curb.

AMBULATION THROUGH DOORWAYS

Door Opens Away from Patient—With Automatic Door Closer The patient approaches the opening edge of the door, and either faces the door directly, or turns sideways to the door with back towards the hinged edge of the door. With the crutches remaining under the axillae) (axillary crutches), or on the forearms (Lofstrand crutches), the patient weight shifts away from the hand that will use the doorknob. The unweighted hand is then placed on the doorknob. Preferably, weight is shifted to the side away from the doorknob, and the hand closest to the doorknob can then be used to open the door.

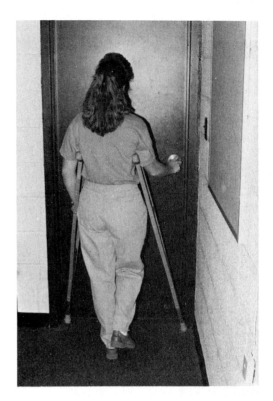

Patient opens door.

Using a quick push, the door is opened wider than is necessary for the patient to move through the doorway. The wider opening of the door is necessitated because the door will start to close automatically until its closing is blocked by the crutches. The hand on the doorknob is quickly returned to the crutch. The crutch tip is placed on the floor between the door and the patient as a doorstop, as close to the opening edge as possible.

Using the crutch tip as a doorstop, the patient steps into the doorway, past the opening edge of the door. As the patient progresses through the doorway, the crutch tip continues to be used as a doorstop.

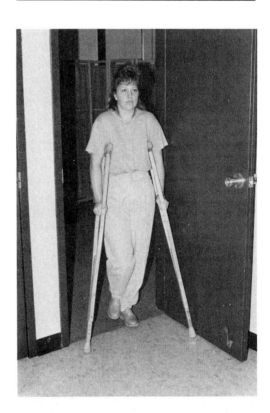

Patient progresses through the doorway, using crutch tip as doorstop.

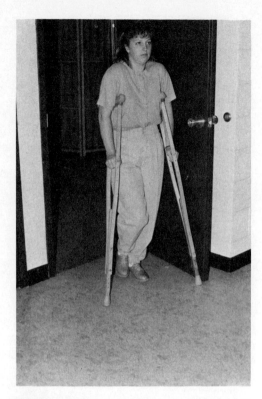

Patient completes passage through the doorway.

After determining that the arc of the closing door will not strike the patient, the patient and crutches complete passage through the doorway, and the door closes automatically.

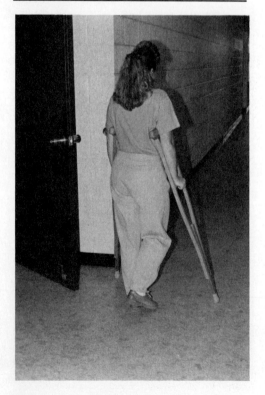

Patient allows door to close.

Door Opens Towards Patient—With Automatic Door Closer The patient approaches the opening edge of the door, standing outside the arc through which the opening door will move. Maintaining the crutches under the axillae (axillary crutches), or on the forearms (Lofstrand crutches), the patient weight shifts to the side away from the hand that will use the doorknob. The unweighted hand is then placed on the doorknob. Preferably, weight is shifted to the side away from the doorknob, and the hand closest to the doorknob can then be used to open the door.

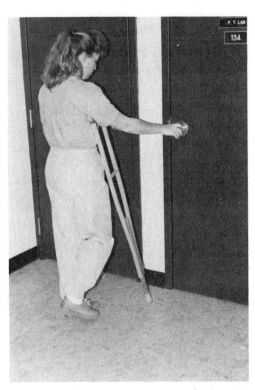

Starting position to open door swinging toward patient.

Using a quick pulling motion, the door is pulled open past the patient, wider than is necessary for the patient to move through the doorway. The wider opening of the door is necessitated because the door will start to close automatically until its closing is blocked by the crutch tip. The hand on the doorknob is quickly returned to the crutch. The crutch tip is placed on the floor as a doorstop between the door and the patient, as close to the opening edge as possible.

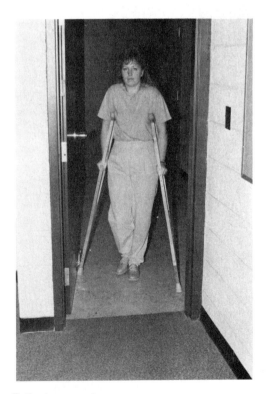

Patient opens door.

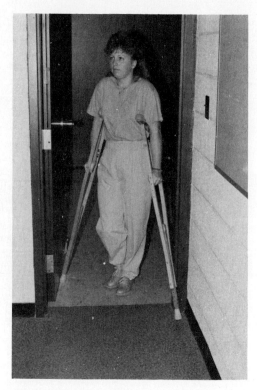

Patient progresses through the doorway, using crutch tip as doorstop.

Maintaining the crutch tip as a doorstop, the patient progresses into the doorway. Stepping through the doorway, the crutch tip, being used as a doorstop, is moved short distances and replaced on the ground quickly to prevent the automatic door closer from causing the door to hit the patient.

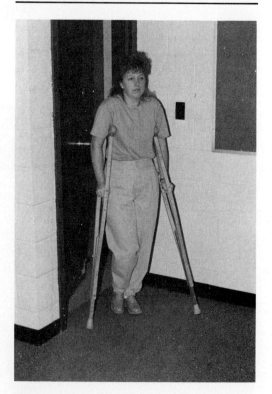

Patient completes passage through the doorway.

Once the patient and crutches have completed passage through the doorway, the door closes automatically.

Without Automatic Door Closer When the door does not have an automatic closer, the initial rapid movement to place the crutch tip on the ground as a doorstop is not necessary. The extra wide opening of the door is also not necessary. Movement of the crutches can be performed more slowly, and placement of the crutch tip as a doorstop between the door and the patient is not required. The patient must turn to close the door because the door will not close automatically.

FOREARM (LOFSTRAND) CRUTCHES

INTRODUCTION

Forearm crutches can be used to perform the three-point, four-point, two-point, swing to, and swing through gait patterns. Patients with marked weakness of both lower extremities, such as a paraplegic patient, would use the swing to or swing through patterns. These patients will use bilateral knee-ankle-foot orthoses (KAFOs), meaning that the patient's knees will be locked in extension and the feet fixed in slight dorsiflexion. Patients may initially use the swing to gait pattern. As ability improves, the patient may progress to the swing through pattern. The swing through gait pattern is more efficient and allows the patient to move faster.

For the purposes of this text, the illustrations of forearm crutches are simulating a paraplegic gait. The subject is assumed to be using KAFOs.

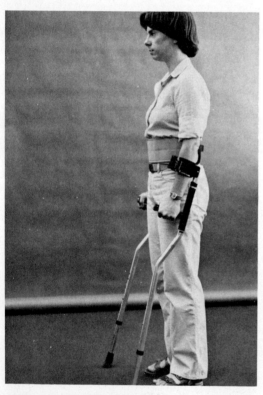

Correct fit of forearm crutches.

FITTING

Forearm crutches are fitting in much the same manner as axillary crutches. The crutch tip is positioned six inches away from the toes at a 45° angle. The handgrip is level with the ulnar styloid process when the arm is relaxed at the side. When the handgrips are held with the shoulders relaxed, the elbows should be in 20° to 30° flexion. The forearm cuff should be as high as possible on the forearm without interfering with full elbow flexion. The cuff should be tight enough to stay on the arm, but loose enough not to bind.

IN AND OUT OF WHEELCHAIR

Two methods may be used to come to standing with forearm crutches and KAFOs. The turn around method requires less strength than the forward method. In both methods the wheelchair is properly positioned and locked. The footrests are removed or pivoted to the side. The patient scoots to the front edge of the wheelchair seat and locks her KAFOs in knee extension. The forearm crutches are placed one on either side of the wheelchair, leaning against the back part of the armrests.

The therapist initially stands slightly behind and to the side away from which the patient will turn. His feet are in stride. One hand grasps the gait belt and the other hand is placed on the patient's shoulder. The therapist must be prepared to move with the patient so as not to inhibit the patient's fluid motion. Initially, the therapist must assist by lifting or guiding the patient.

If the patient is to pivot to her left, she begins by crossing her right leg over her left leg by hooking the medial upright of the right orthosis over the medial upright of the left orthosis. This aids in placement of the legs as the patient turns. The patient then pivots onto the side to which she will turn.

The patient reaches behind her with her left hand and grasps the right armrest. Her right hand reaches in front and grasps the left armrest.

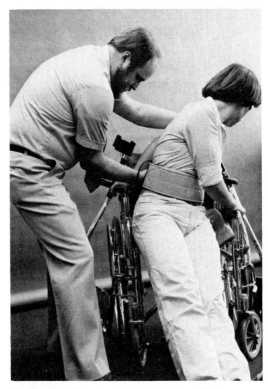

Starting position to get out of wheelchair; turn around method.

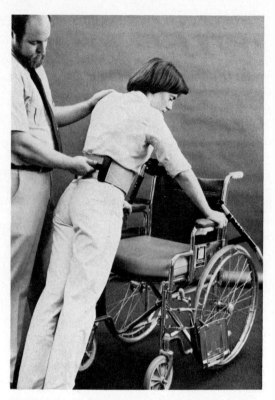

Pushing to standing while completing the turn.

She then pushes to standing, completing the turn as she attains the standing position.

Holding onto the armrest, the patient pulls her feet closer to the wheelchair. The patient shifts her weight to one side and picks up the forearm crutch on the other side.

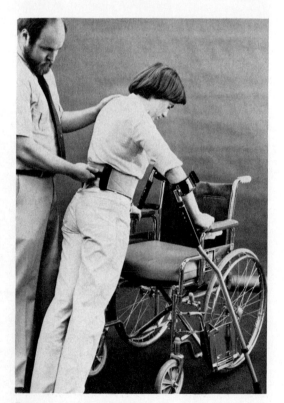

Retrieving and positioning one crutch.

The patient pushes to the fully upright position, keeping her shoulders behind her hips in order to maintain hip extension. This posture is called a "C" curve. The patient backs up to move away from the wheelchair.

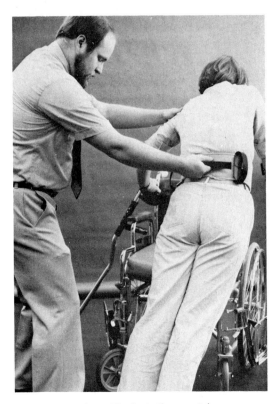

Retrieving and positioning other crutch.

Placing her weight on the single forearm crutch, the patient removes her other hand from the armrest. She then picks up the second forearm crutch and places it properly.

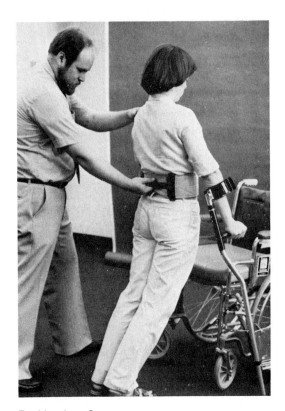

Pushing into C curve.

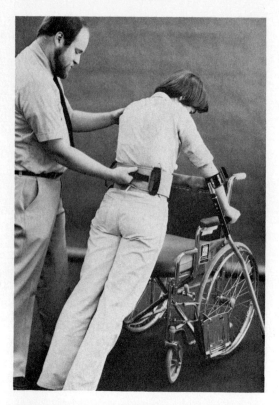

Starting position for sitting; turn around method.

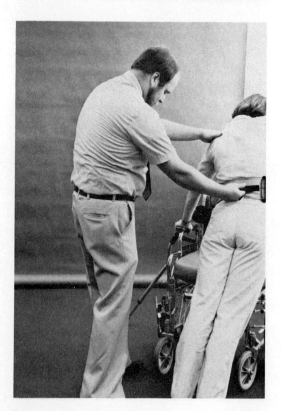

Removing one crutch.

To sit down using the turn around method, the patient walks to the wheelchair. The patient faces the wheelchair with the crutches spread on either side of the wheelchair. The wheelchair is properly positioned, locked, and the footrests are moved out of the way.

The therapist stands slightly behind and on the side to which the patient will turn. His feet are in stride. One hand grasps the gait belt and the other hand is placed on the patient's shoulders. The therapist must be prepared to move as the patient moves in order to avoid interfering with the patient's fluid motion. Initially, the therapist may control the rate at which the patient turns and sits.

The patient shifts her weight to one forearm crutch, and then removes the other forearm crutch. The crutch that has been removed is placed against the armrest. Then the patient grasps the armrest with her free hand.

The patient shifts her weight onto the armrest and removes the remaining crutch, placing it against the armrest. She is then able to grasp the other armrest.

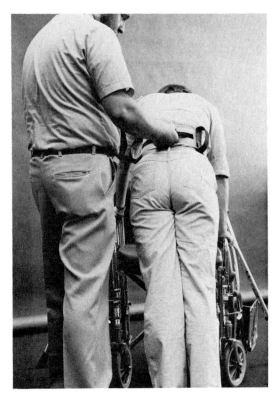

Removing other crutch.

The patient pivots, lowering herself into the chair. Repositioning her arm, the patient can unlock the knee locks on the KAFOs, readjust her position, and place her feet on the footrests.

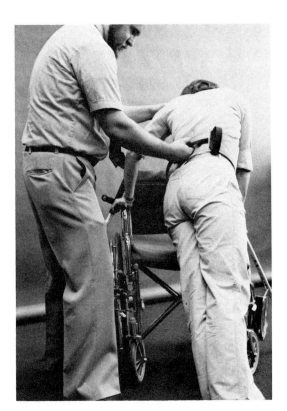

Beginning the turn and lowering to seat.

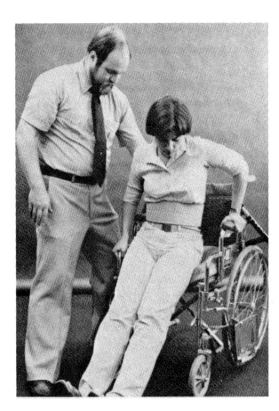

Completing assumption of sitting posture.

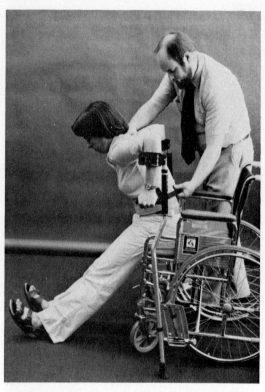

Starting position to get out of wheelchair; forward method.

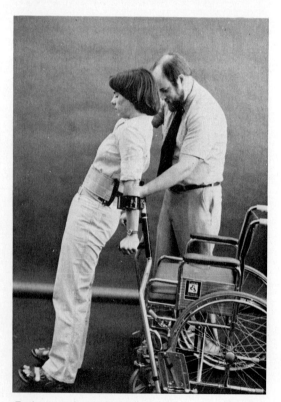

Patient pushes to standing.

In preparation for the forward method of getting out of the wheelchair, the wheelchair is properly positioned, locked, and the footrests are moved out of the way. The patient scoots to the front edge of the seat and locks the knee locks on the KAFOs. Grasping the crutches, the patient places the crutch tips approximately even with the hips.

The therapist stands slightly behind and to one side of the patient. One hand grasps the gait belt and the other hand is placed on the patient's shoulder. His feet are in stride to allow him to move as the patient moves.

The patient pushes on the crutches, extending her arms and depressing her shoulders in order to raise her body. The movement must be a quick thrust so that the body is propelled upward and forward. The therapist may assist by lifting and pushing the patient forward.

The crutches are brought forward quickly to halt the forward momentum of the patient's body. The therapist can assist the patient into the arched position necessary to maintain standing by pushing forward on the gait belt and pulling backward on the shoulder (see top photo).

Prior to the patient sitting down, the wheelchair is positioned, locked, and the footrests are moved out of the way. To sit, the patient backs up to the wheelchair. The patient moves her crutches backward, placing the tips even with the center of the seat on either side of wheelchair. She then lowers herself into the wheelchair by flexing her arms and upper trunk.

The therapist stands slightly behind and to one side, with one hand on the gait belt and the other hand on the shoulder. His feet are in stride. The therapist may assist by controlling the rate of sitting.

The patient removes the crutches and unlocks the knee locks on her KAFOs. She can then readjust the footrests and her position in the wheelchair.

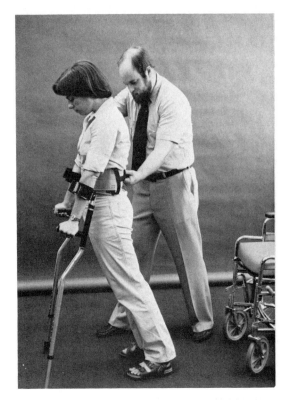

Crutches are repositioned quickly; C curve is attained.

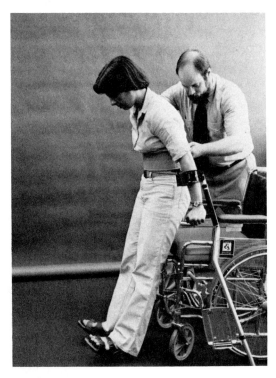

Initiating sitting down.

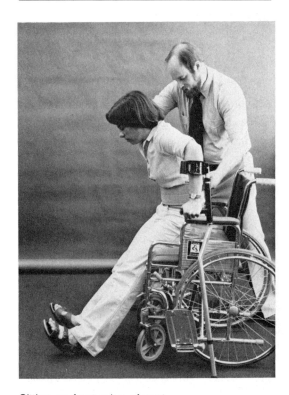

Sitting on front edge of seat.

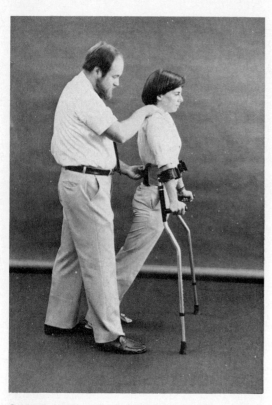

Starting position; swing-to gait pattern.

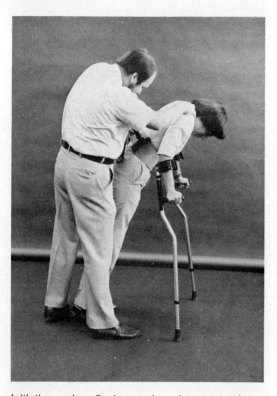

Initiating swing, flexing neck and upper trunk
while depressing shoulders and extending arms.

SWING-TO GAIT PATTERN

In the starting position, the patient's hips are maintained in extension by keeping her shoulders behind her hips. The therapist can assist in maintaining the C curve by pushing forward with the hand on the gait belt while pulling backward with the hand on the shoulder. His feet are in stride as he stands behind and slightly to one side of the patient.

To initiate the swing-to gait pattern, the crutches are advanced approximately one stride length in front of the patient's toes.

To lift her body, the patient extends her arms while pushing down on the crutches. She slightly flexes her trunk in order to lift her feet off the ground. The therapist assists by lifting with the hand on the gait belt.

With her feet off the ground and her trunk flexed, the patient's legs will swing forward because of the pull of gravity. As her legs swing forward, the patient must extend her neck and trunk to regain the C curve. As her feet land in a position parallel to the crutches, the patient's hips must continue to move forward of the shoulders. The therapist assists by pushing with the hand on the gait belt and pulling backward with the hand on the patient's shoulder.

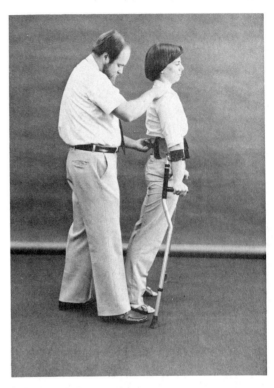

Swinging to the crutches.

Once the C curve is regained, the crutches are advanced. The sequence is repeated for continued progression.

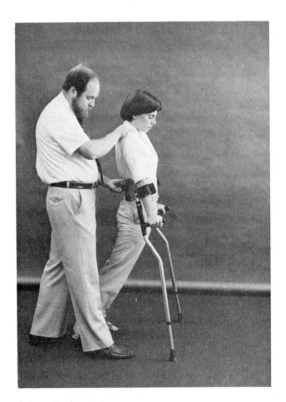

Advancing crutches.

SWING-THROUGH GAIT PATTERN

The starting position and trunk movements are the same as for the swing-to gait pattern. However, in this case, the patient allows her legs to swing beyond the crutches as she lands. Thus the crutches and feet do not end up in one line. Because of the momentum generated by the larger swing, the crutches must be brought forward quickly to keep the patient from falling forward.

The role and position of the therapist remain the same.

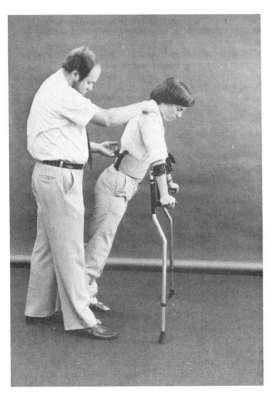

Starting position; swing-through gait pattern.

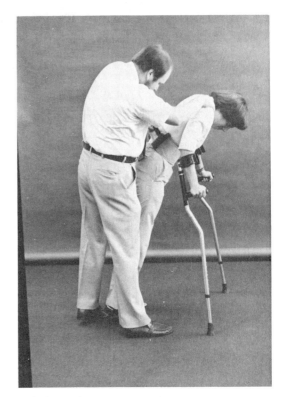

Initiating swing.

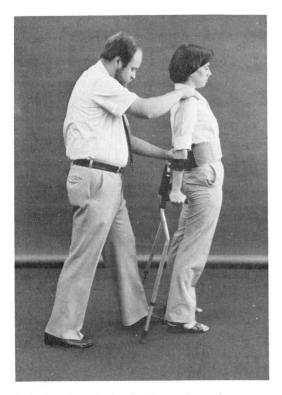

Swinging through; landing beyond crutches.

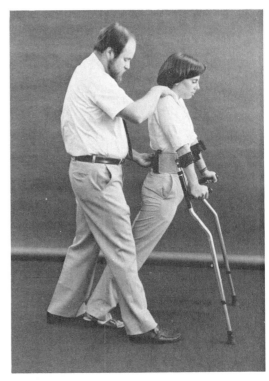

Crutches are advanced quickly to maintain balance.

FALLING

Should the patient start to fall, the therapist must decide to prevent the fall or to control the fall. The usual manner of falling for the paraplegic patient is to lose the C curve and to jack-knife into full hip flexion.

If the therapist decides to prevent the fall, he must be in stride, and close enough to the patient to pull the patient to him. The therapist must then assist the patient back into the C curve by lifting the upper trunk backwards and pushing forward on the gait belt.

If the therapist is going to control the fall and lower the patient to the floor, the patient is instructed to drop her crutches, pushing them slightly away so she does not fall directly on top of them. The patient reaches out to catch herself on slightly flexed arms to absorb the shock of falling without injury to her arms. The therapist assists by controlling the rate of the fall.

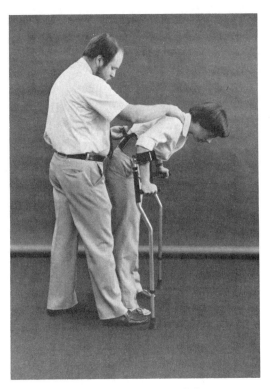

Patient loses C curve; begins to fall.

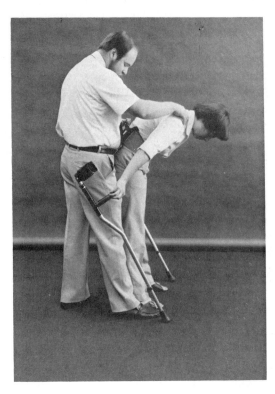

Patient drops crutches to side.

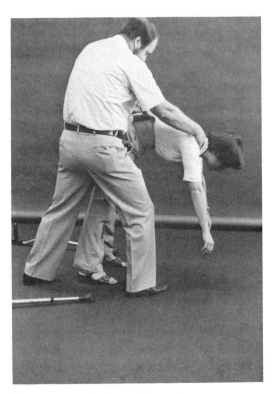

Patient prepares to catch herself.

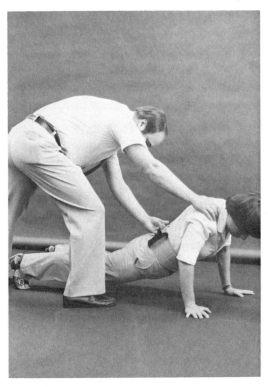

Patient catches herself; absorbs shock by flexing arms.

GETTING UP FROM THE FLOOR

Getting up from the floor is a difficult maneuver. The easiest method is to crawl to a chair or other sturdy object, and pull up using the object as a support. Other methods of getting up from the floor are described in chapter 8 (see pages 209 to 219).

First, the patient retrieves her crutches. They are positioned with the tips towards her feet and with the tips approximately at the level of her knees.

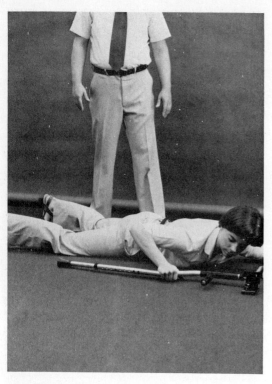

Preparing to get up from floor; positioning crutches.

Grasping one crutch and placing it upright, she places the other hand on the floor. She then pushes up with the hand on the floor and pulls up with the hand on the crutch. The therapist stands in stride to one side, placing one hand on the gait belt and the other hand on the patient's shoulder. He can assist by lifting with the hand on the gait belt.

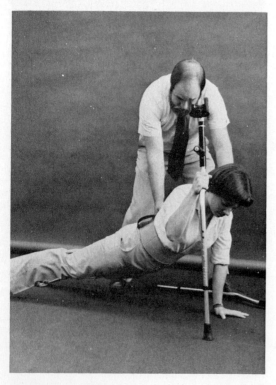

Pushing up from floor.

The patient must grasp the handgrip of the crutch while balancing on the hand on the floor. The therapist can assist the patient to maintain her balance.

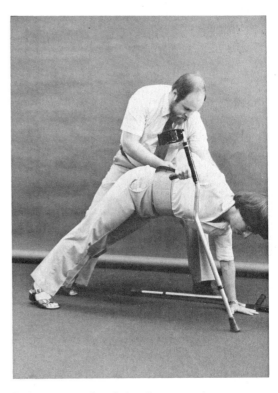

Patient grasps handgrip of one crutch.

The patient's weight is then shifted and balanced on the crutch. This leaves the other hand free to grasp the remaining crutch.

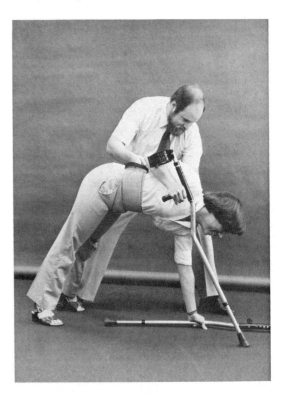

Patient grasps other crutch.

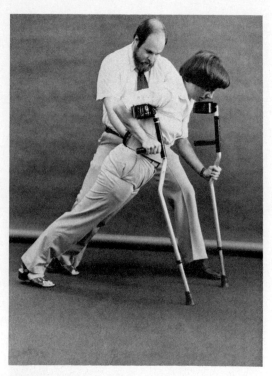

Patient pushes to upright position.

The second crutch is positioned upright with the tip parallel to the first crutch. The patient then pushes to the C curve position using both crutches.

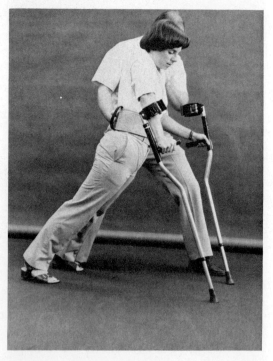

Positioning crutches properly.

The crutches are properly positioned one at a time, and the patient is ready to ambulate.

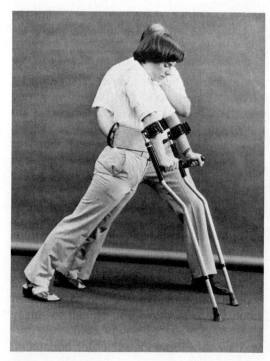

Ready to ambulate.

STAIRS

There are two basic methods for ambulation on the stairs; the forward and the backward methods. In each case, the same sequence may be used to ascend or descend curbs. In either case, the patient can use one stair rail and one crutch, or she can use two crutches. It is usually easier to teach the patient initially to use one crutch and one stair rail. If this method is used, the second crutch must be carried also so it is available when the top, or bottom, of the stairs is reached. The crutch may be carried in either hand.

To ascend the stairs using the forward method, the patient starts in the C curve position facing the stairs. The feet and crutch tips are parallel at the base of the first stair. The therapist stands behind the patient in stride, grasping the gait belt with one hand while the other hand grasps the stair rail.

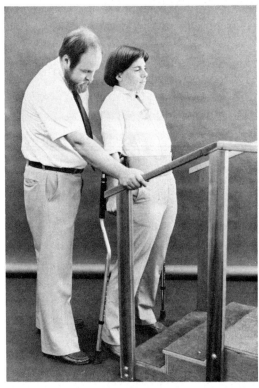

Starting position to ascend stairs; forward method.

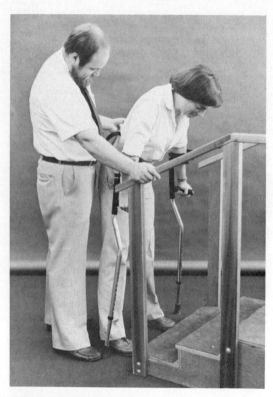

Initiating raising the body.

The patient uses the same neck, upper trunk, and arm motions used during ambulation. Flexing the neck and upper trunk, she extends her arms and depresses her shoulders to raise her body. This lifts the patient's feet off the ground, allowing her to place them on the next higher stair. As she places her feet, the patient extends her neck and trunk to regain the C curve. Momentum contributes to the success of this maneuver, so it must be performed rapidly. The crutches are advanced to the same stair as the feet.

The therapist assists by lifting on the gait belt as the patient raises her body. He may also assist the patient in regaining the C curve by pushing forward on the gait belt and pulling back on the patient's shoulder.

The sequence is repeated to ascend the entire flight of stairs.

Initially, this maneuver may require the assistance of two people to ensure patient safety.

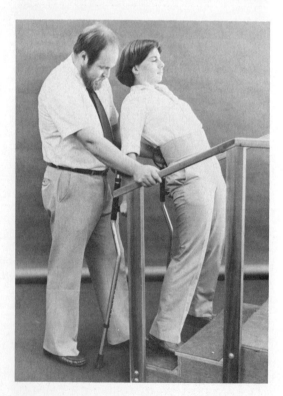

Patient advances both feet to same stair simultaneously.

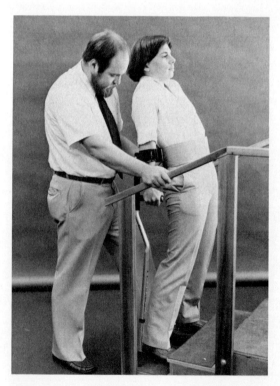

Both crutches are advanced to same stair.

To descend the stairs using the forward method, the patient is at the top of the stairs facing down the stairs. The therapist is on the stairs in front of the patient. He stands in stride, grasping the gait belt and the stair rail.

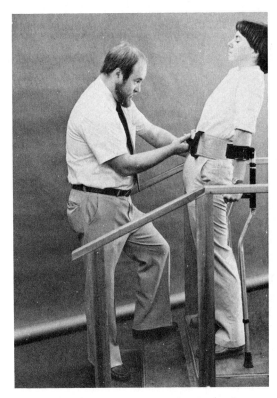

Starting position to descend stairs; forward method.

The same neck, upper trunk, and arm motions used in ambulating are used to raise the body. The feet are lowered to the next stair first, and then the crutches are brought quickly to the same stair to regain balance in the C curve. The therapist must stay close enough to the patient for guarding, but not be so close as to interfere with the patient's freedom of movement.

The sequence is repeated to descend the remaining stairs.

The patient may often descend several steps at one time.

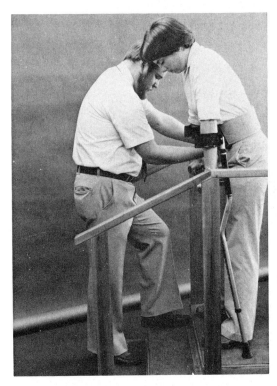

Initiating raising of the body.

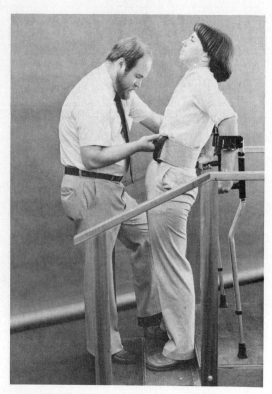

Patient lowers both feet to same stair simultaneously.

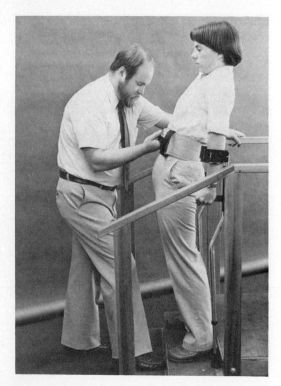

Both crutches are lowered to same stair.

Ascending the stairs using the backward method requires that the patient face away from the stairs. The feet and crutch tips are parallel to the base of the first stair, with the crutches slightly behind the patient's feet. The therapist is in front of the patient in a stride position, facing up the stairs. He grasps the gait belt and stair rail.

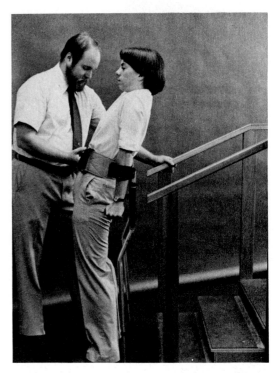

Starting position to ascend stairs; backward method.

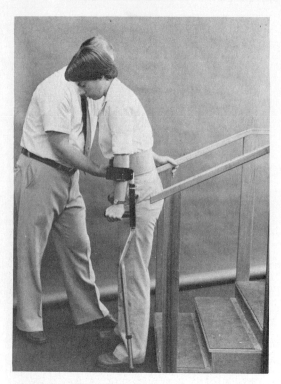

Initiating raising of the body.

Again, the same neck, upper trunk, and arm motions used in ambulating are used to raise the patient's body. As the patient raises her body, her legs are allowed to swing backward onto the first stair. The patient must immediately extend her neck and upper trunk in order to regain the C curve. The crutches are brought to the same stair. The therapist may assist in placement of the legs by pushing on the gait belt and regaining of the C curve by pulling on the gait belt.

The sequence is repeated to ascend the remaining stairs.

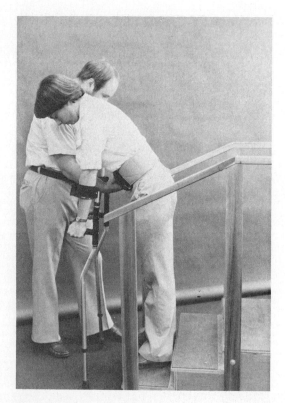

Patient places both feet on one stair simultaneously.

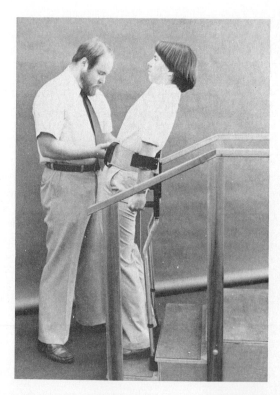

Both crutches are placed on same stair as feet.

The starting position of descending the stairs using the backward method requires the patient to stand at the top of the stairs facing away from the stairs. The crutch tips are parallel to the first stair, and are slightly behind the patient's feet. The patient maintains the C curve. The therapist stands on the stairs in stride, behind the patient. One hand grasps the gait belt and the other hand grasps the stair rail.

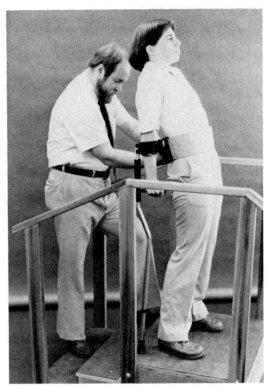

Starting position to descend stairs; backward method.

The same neck, upper trunk, and arm motions used in ambulating are used to raise the patient's body. As the patient raises her body, her feet swing backward over the next lower step. She then lowers herself to that step and immediately regains the C curve. The crutch tips are then placed on the same step. The therapist assists the lift by lifting on the gait belt and assists regaining the C curve by pushing on the gait belt.

The sequence is repeated to descend the remaining stairs.

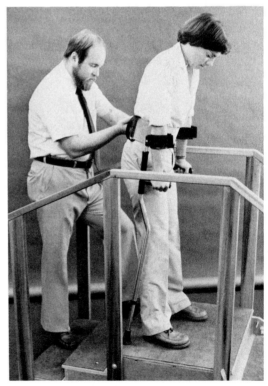

Initiating raising of the body.

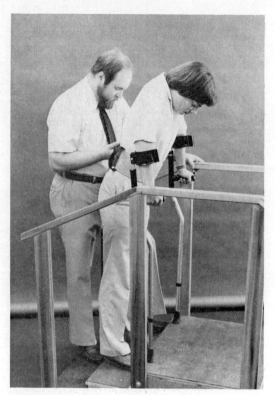

Patient lowers both feet to same stair simultaneously.

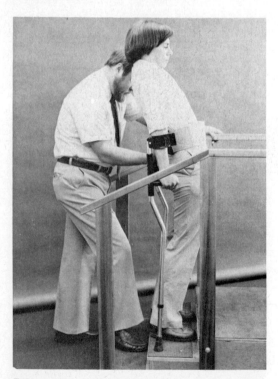

Both crutches are placed on same stair as feet.

CANES

INTRODUCTION

Canes provide the least amount of support of the assistive devices used for gait. One or two canes may be used for balance or to relieve weight bearing on a lower extremity. When one cane is used to relieve weight bearing, it is initially placed on the side opposite to the involved lower extremity. This placement allows the patient's weight to be shifted towards the stronger side by increasing the base of support on the stronger side. Later, when weight bearing on the involved lower extremity is desired, the cane can be moved to the hand on the involved side.

FITTING

With the cane alongside the toes, the top of the cane should be aligned with the patient's ulnar styloid process. This allows 20° to 30° elbow flexion when the cane is held properly. When used properly, the force on the cane should be exerted directly downward.

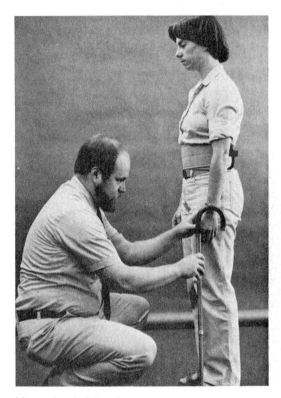

Measuring height of cane.

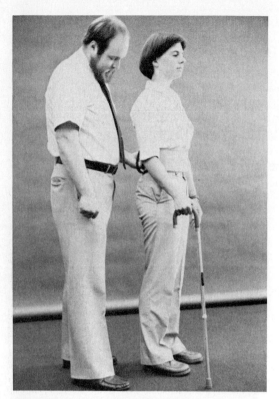

Correct manner of grasping cane.

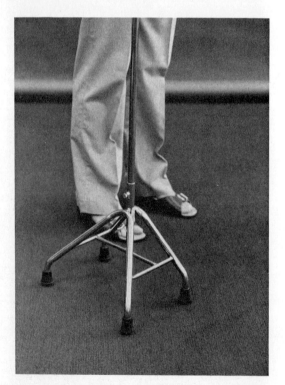

Correct orientation for quad cane.

When using a quad cane, the longer legs of the quad cane are positioned away from the patient. This reduces the risk of the patient catching her foot on the legs of the cane. The quad cane is measured and used in the same manner as the standard cane.

IN AND OUT OF WHEELCHAIR

In the following examples of moving in and out of the wheelchair using a cane, the patient is role playing greater strength on one side, such as might be observed in a patient with hemiplegia. A patient who has the use of both arms would place both hands on the respective armrests to assist raising or lowering.

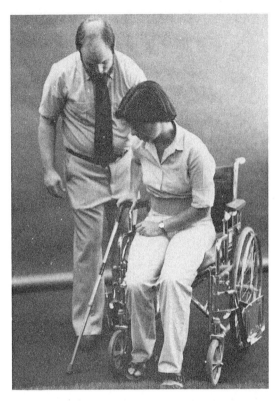

Preparing to stand; using standard cane.

Before starting, the wheelchair must be properly positioned, locked, and the footrests removed or pivoted out of the way. The patient scoots to the front edge of the seat. When using a standard cane, the patient holds the cane in her hand as she grasps the armrest. The patient's feet are placed on the floor together or in stride, close to the front edge of the wheelchair seat. Initiating the movement with trunk flexion, the patient pushes to standing using one or both arms. If two canes are used, one cane is grasped in each hand as the patient grasps the armrests.

The therapist stands slightly behind and to the side of the patient with the cane. One hand grasps the gait belt and the other hand is placed on the patient's shoulder.

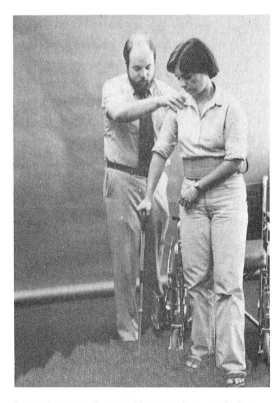

Assuming standing position; ready to ambulate.

To return to sitting, the patient walks to the wheelchair and checks that it is properly positioned, locked, and the footrests are out of the way. The patient then turns and backs up until the front edge of the wheelchair seat is felt at the backs of the knees. Reaching back with one arm at a time, the patient grasps the armrests and lowers herself into the wheelchair. She can then secure the cane and adjust the footrests and her position in the wheelchair.

The therapist remains in the same relative position throughout ambulation, and moving in and out of the wheelchair. He can assist by controlling balance, turning, and lowering into the wheelchair.

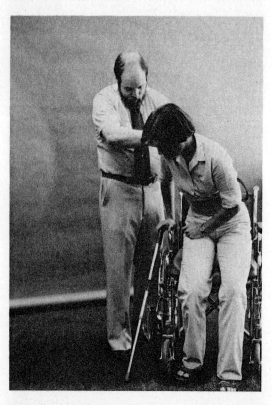

Lowering to sitting.

When a quad cane is used, the quad cane is positioned slightly in front and to the side of the patient. The patient moves to standing by pushing with her strong hand on the armrest. Once standing, she grasps the quad cane. The therapist's position is behind and slightly to The side of the patient.

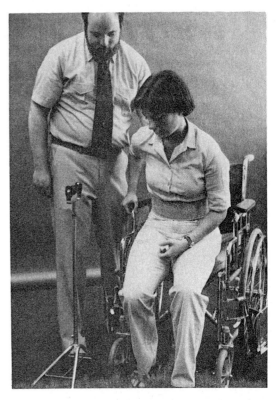

Preparing to stand; using quad cane.

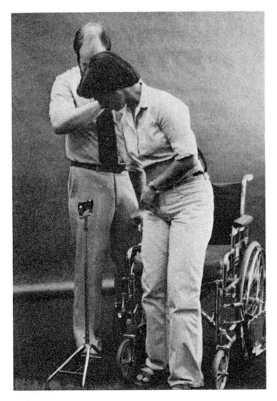

Pushing to standing using armrest.

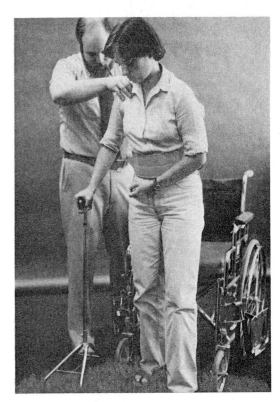

Grasping quad cane; ready to ambulate.

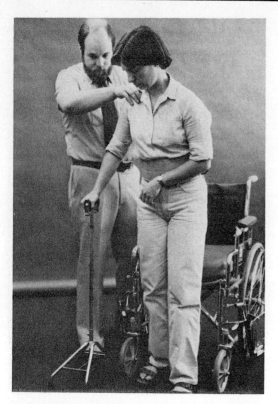

Preparing to sit; using a quad cane.

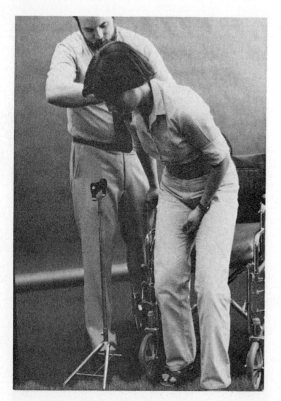

Lowering to sitting using armrest.

To sit when using a quad cane, the patient faces away from the wheelchair, releases the quad cane, and reaches for the armrest. While grasping the armrest, the patient lowers herself into the wheelchair. The therapist stands in stride behind and to one side of the patient.

AMBULATION WITH ONE CANE

In the starting position, the patient's feet are parallel and the cane is next to the small toe. The therapist stands behind and slightly to the side. One hand grasps the gait belt and the other hand is placed on the patient's shoulder.

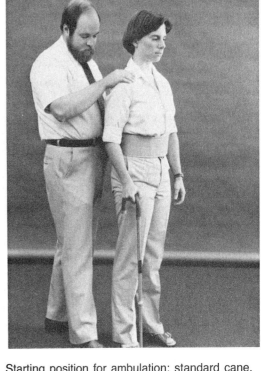

Starting position for ambulation; standard cane.

The cane is advanced first, approximately one stride length ahead. The therapist steps forward with his outside foot.

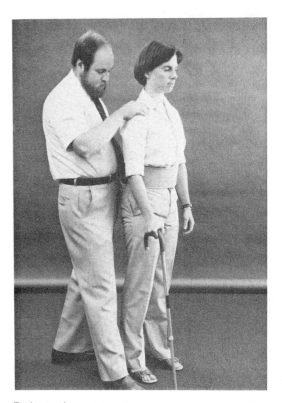

Patient advances cane.

The patient advances the foot opposite to the cane up to the cane.

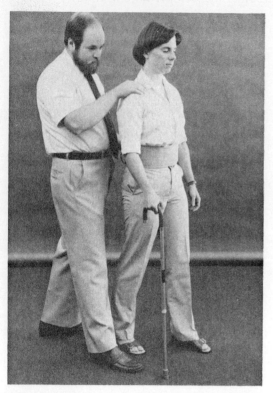

Patient advances foot opposite cane up to cane.

The patient then advances her other foot. Initially, the patient may only step to the other foot and cane. The patient should be encouraged to step beyond the other foot and cane in order to develop a more normal rhythm and gait pattern. The therapist advances his inside foot as the patient steps through.

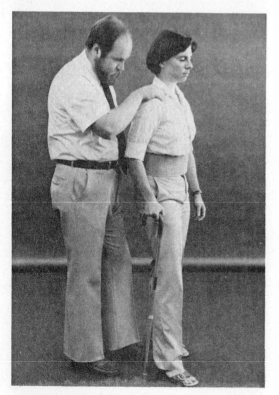

Patient steps past cane with other foot.

STAIRS WITH ONE CANE

Initially, the patient should be taught to use the stair rail for more stability. If the patient has been using the cane in her right hand when ambulating on level surfaces, she may switch the cane to her left hand, or she may hold the cane and stair rail with her right hand. This will allow her to ascend and descend on the right, as is customary. If the patient is unable to use her right hand, she can ascend on the left, holding the stair rail with her left hand.

The sequence for ascending and descending stairs may also be used to ascend and descend curbs.

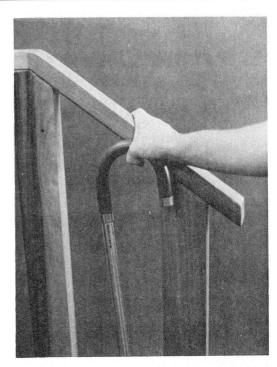

One method of holding cane in hand grasping stair rail.

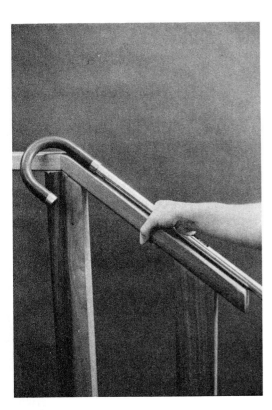

Second method of holding cane in hand grasping stair rail.

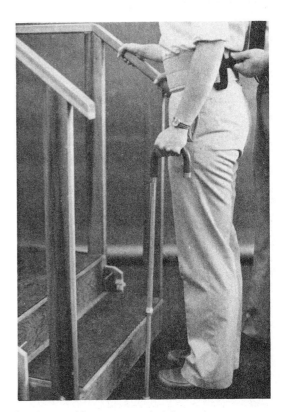

Starting position to ascend stairs; using cane and stair rail.

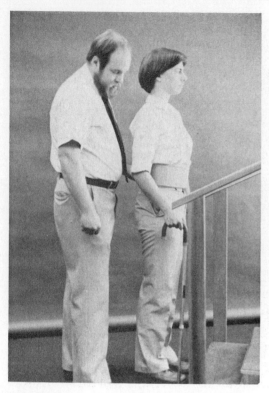

Starting position to ascend stairs; using one cane.

The starting position for ascending stairs requires that the patient face the stairs. The feet and cane are parallel to the base of the first stair. The therapist stands behind the patient, grasping the gait belt and the stair rail.

The stronger leg is placed on the next higher stair.

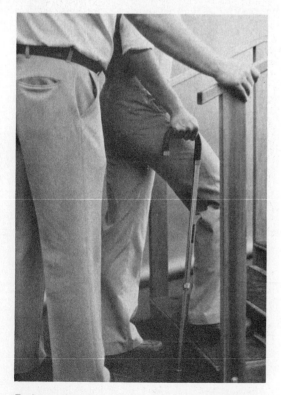

Patient advances stronger leg to next stair.

By extending the stronger leg, the patient raises her body and places the involved lower extremity on the same stair as the stronger leg. The cane may be advanced at the same time as the involved extremity, or separately. The cane is placed midway between the front and back of the stair tread.

The therapist remains in stride behind the patient.

The sequence is repeated to ascend the remaining stairs.

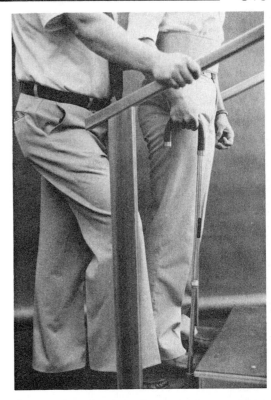

Cane and weaker leg advanced to same stair.

To descend the stairs, the patient faces the stairs, standing with her feet and cane parallel to the top step. The therapist stands in stride on the stairs, facing the patient. He grasps the gait belt with one hand and the stair rail with the other hand.

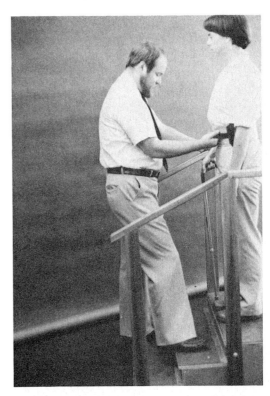

Starting position to descend stairs; using one cane.

The involved lower extremity and cane are lowered to the next lower step by having the patient slowly flex the stronger leg. As the cane is moved to the next lower step, it should be placed two thirds of the way forward on the stair tread.

Once this has been accomplished, the stronger leg is lowered to the same step. The therapist remains in stride, moving to avoid interfering with the patient's movement.

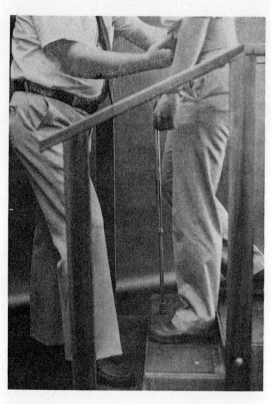

Patient lowers involved leg and cane at same time.

AMBULATION WITH TWO CANES—THREE-POINT GAIT PATTERN

To ambulate using two canes in the three-point gait pattern, the canes are placed on the floor approximately 6 inches away from the toes at a 45° angle. They are parallel to each other, as are the patient's feet. The therapist stands behind and slightly to one side of the patient. One hand grasps the gait belt and the other hand is placed on the patient's shoulder.

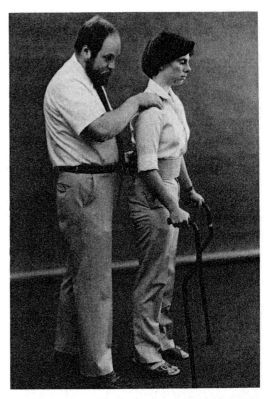

Starting position for ambulation; two canes; three-point gait pattern.

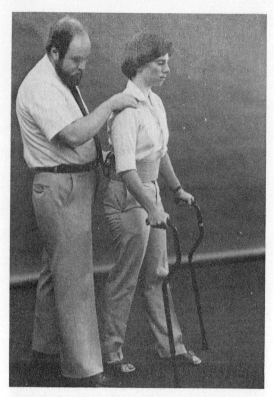

Patient advances both cane and involved leg.

Both canes and the involved lower extremity are advanced at the same time approximately one stride length. The patient may initially advance the canes first and then the involved lower extremity until she is comfortable with the gait pattern. The therapist moves his outside, or right, leg forward.

The patient then bears weight on the canes, and moves the stronger leg forward beyond the line of the canes and involved lower extremity. The therapist steps forward with his inside, or left, foot.

The sequence is repeated for continued progression.

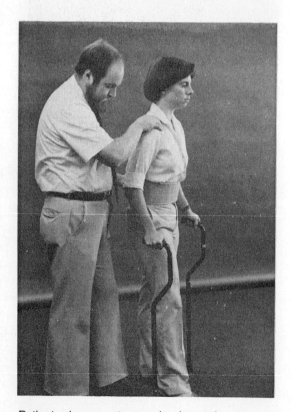

Patient advances stronger leg beyond cane.

AMBULATION WITH TWO CANES—FOUR-POINT GAIT PATTERN

The starting position for ambulation with two canes in a four-point gait is the same as for the three-point gait for both the patient and the therapist.

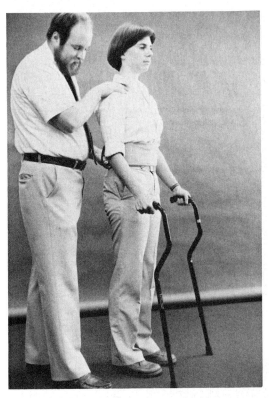

Starting position for ambulation; two canes; four-point gait pattern.

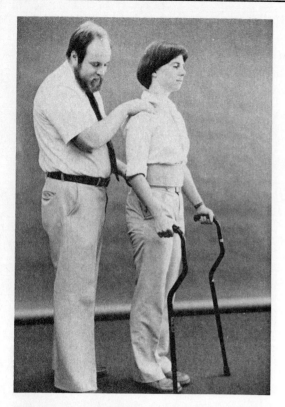

Patient advances left cane.

Each cane and lower extremity is moved separately. In this series of four illustrations, the left cane is advanced first.

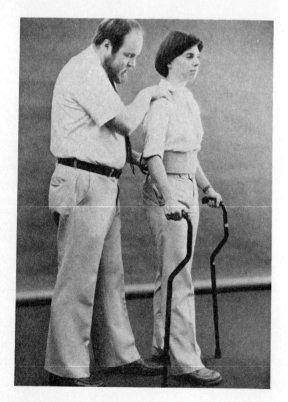

Patient advances right foot.

The right foot is advanced to the same line as the left cane. The therapist's inside, or left, foot is advanced forward.

The patient advances the right cane a normal stride length. The therapist advances his outside, or right, foot.

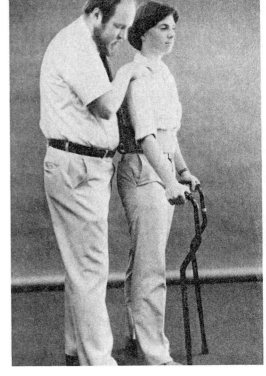

Patient advances right cane.

The patient's left foot is advanced to a line even with the right cane.

The sequence is repeated for continued progression.

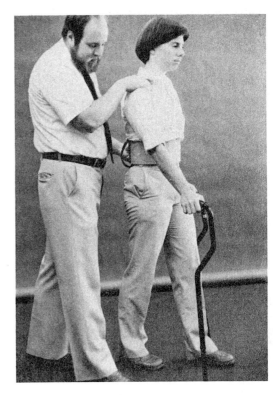

Patient advances left foot.

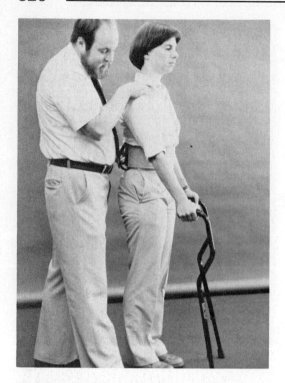

Starting position for ambulation; two canes; two-point gait pattern.

AMBULATION WITH TWO CANES— TWO-POINT GAIT PATTERN

The starting position is the same as for the three-point gait pattern for both the patient and the therapist. In this sequence of illustrations, the left cane and the patient's right foot are advanced at the same time. The therapist advances his inside, or left, foot.

Once this has been accomplished, the patient advances the right cane and her left foot a normal stride length. The therapist advances his outside, or right, foot.

The sequence is repeated for continued progression.

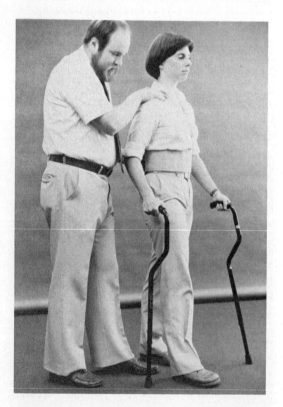

Patient advances left cane and right foot at same time.

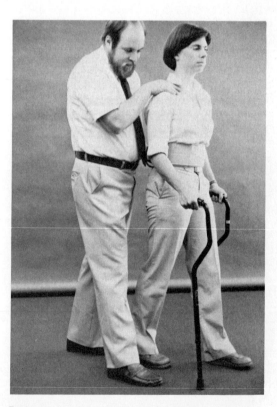

Patient advances right cane and left foot at same time.

STAIRS WITH TWO CANES

One method of ascending and descending stairs with two canes requires the same starting position and maneuvers for both patient and therapist that are illustrated on pages 317 through 320. The only difference is that either both canes are held in one hand while the other hand grasps the stair rail, or one cane is used while the other cane is held in the hand that is grasping the stair rail. The top photo illustrates the method of holding both canes in one hand while grasping the stair rail with the other hand.

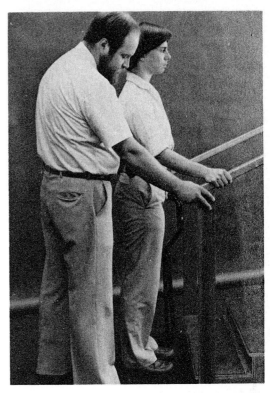

Preparing to ascend stairs; both canes in left hand.

The other commonly used method of using two canes on the stairs is to use one cane in each hand. In the starting position for using two canes to ascend stairs, the patient is facing the stairs with both feet and canes parallel to the base of the first stair. The therapist stands in stride behind the patient, with one hand grasping the gait belt and the other hand grasping the stair rail.

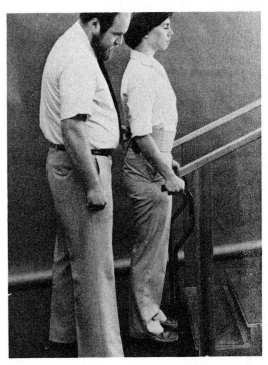

Starting position to ascend stairs; using two canes.

The patient advances the stronger leg to the next higher stair.

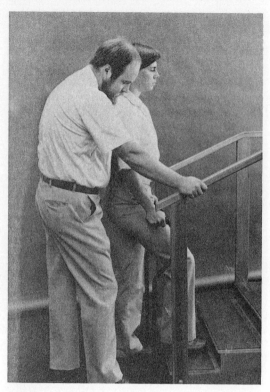

Patient advances stronger leg to next higher stair.

The stronger leg is used to raise the body so both canes and the weaker leg can be placed on the same stair. The canes and weaker leg can advance together, or the leg and then the canes can advance separately. The canes should be placed midway from front to back on the stair tread. The therapist remains in stride behind the patient throughout the sequence.

The sequence is repeated to ascend the remaining stairs.

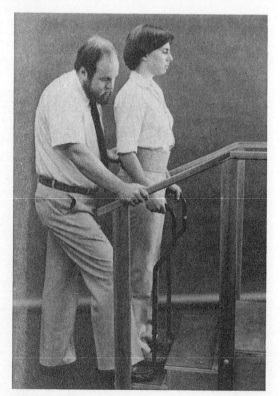

Patient advances both canes and involved leg to same stair at same time.

To descend the stairs using the two canes without a stair rail, the patient stands with her feet and canes parallel to the top step, facing down the stairs. The therapist stands in stride on the stairs, facing the patient. One hand grasps the gait belt and the other hand grasps the stair rail.

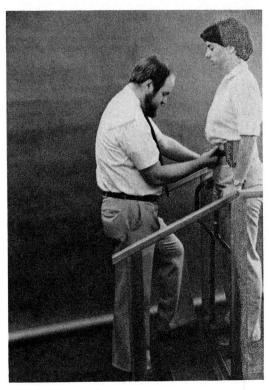

Starting position to descend stairs; using two canes.

By slowly flexing her stronger leg, the patient lowers the involved leg and both canes to the next lower stair. The canes and involved leg may be lowered together, or the involved leg may be lowered separately from the canes.

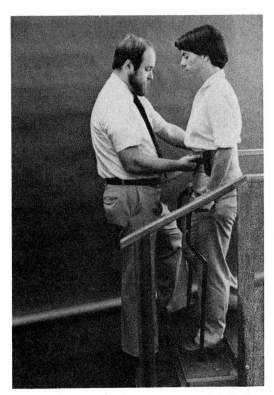

Patient lowers both canes and involved leg at same time.

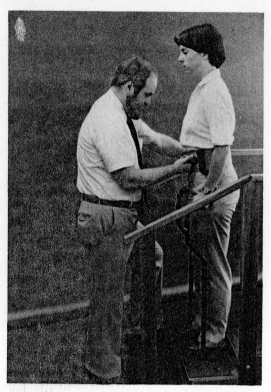

Patient lowers stronger leg to same stair as canes.

While bearing weight on the canes, the patient then lowers the stronger leg to the same stair as the canes and the involved leg. The therapist remains in stride in front of the patient, moving to avoid interfering with the patient's movement.

The sequence is repeated to descend the remaining stairs.

The same sequence may be used to ascend or descend a curb.

AMBULATION THROUGH DOORWAYS

Ambulation through doorways with canes follows the same sequence as ambulation through doorways with crutches. In many cases, the process with canes will be easier than with crutches because canes are lighter and not as unwieldy as crutches. Also, a patient using canes usually has a more advanced capability of balance and ambulation than does a patient who must use crutches.